Handbook of Psychological Signs, Symptoms, and Syndromes

Donald P. Ogdon, Ph.D., F.S.P.A.
Old Dominion University
Eastern Virginia Medical School

Published by

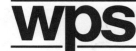

WESTERN PSYCHOLOGICAL SERVICES
Publishers and Distributors
12031 Wilshire Boulevard
Los Angeles, California 90025-1251

Library of Congress Catalog Card Number: 81-52961
International Standard Book Number: 0-87424-173-1

Fifth Printing .... October 1993

To the memory of my parents
Glenn H. Ogdon (1893-1980)
Elizabeth McDonald Ogdon (1899-1977)

TABLE OF CONTENTS

PREFACE

The requirements for appropriate use of this book are the same as those cited in *Psychodiagnostics and Personality Assessment: A Handbook* (2nd ed.) (Ogdon, 1975). Students and interns would do well to review those. Briefly, the user should have an understanding of and compentency in the fields of clinical psychology, including personality theory, and abnormal psychology. Furthermore, the user should be thoroughly familiar with projective psychology and psychological tests.

Many of the individual test signs presented here are part of scales or constellations of signs. These should be used in concert for maximum effectiveness. Test indices included here also vary along the five dimensions described in Ogdon (1975, p. 4), and reference to them is also encouraged for a full appreciation of the use of signs in the assessment process.

A preliminary attempt was made to evaluate the relative value of each sign for each condition, symptom, or syndrome. It became apparent rather quickly that the currently available data do not readily lend themselves to such an evaluation. Such a rigorous evaluation must await clarification by further study and research.

The reader will note that a significant feature of this text is the uniform organization of each section. In each instance, a condition, symptom, or syndrome is first defined and delineated. Then behavioral signs of each are presented. These are followed by Wechsler, Rorschach, projective drawing, and Bender-Gestalt signs, consecutively. In a few cases, a particular test may yield no indices of a particular condition. In those instances, of course, no reference is made to that test. Finally, most sections conclude with a presentation of contraindications for the condition under consideration. This format facilitates rapid location of data pertaining to any particular set of test data for each condition or syndrome addressed.

The discussions of behavioral manifestations of some psychological trait or condition are set apart from the test indices of the trait or condition as a matter of convenience of presentation. This certainly should not be considered as an indication that the author feels the test signs are not "behavioral manifestations." Of course they are. A more accurate depiction of these behavioral manifestations would be "behavior associated with a given personality condition or characteristic that is not formally considered a response to a particular test." This more accurate description was deemed too wordy and unnecessarily elaborate for use throughout this volume, so we opted for the shorter expression.

The selection of the four psychological tests used in the discussions of test indices follows essentially the same reasoning put forth in Ogdon (1975) and need not be reiterated here. Publications by Crenshaw, Bohn, Hoffman, Matheus, and Offenbach (1968), Fein (1979), Lubin, Wallis, and Paine (1971), and Sundberg (1961) contain the gist of the reasons for selecting these particular psychological tests with which to work. Except for Fein (1979), these publications are considered in greater detail in Ogdon (1975).

For individuals with limited experience with Rorschach's test, Exner's volumes (1974, 1978) provide many useful responses along with sample protocols. For those with limited experience with projective drawings, Wenck's (1977) handbook contains nearly a hundred pages of illustrations of diagnostic signs for the House-Tree-Person Test (H-T-P). Hutt's (1977) text gives numerous examples of Bender-Gestalt reproductions of individuals with various conditions and diagnoses. While these are not an altogether satisfactory substitute for actual clinical experience with the tests, they do provide a wide variety of response manifestations which should be quite helpful to the psychologist in training.

One cannot complete a book of this type without a little help from his friends. Graduate students of mine made contributions by searching library stacks for references and I am very grateful for their help. Lindsay Gibson, in particular, was most helpful in this regard. Proofreading is more onerous than library searching. Michael Nahl and Shirley Taylor worked far into the night on this chore and also made numerous editorial suggestions which are sincerely appreciated. The help of all those students and friends is gratefully appreciated.

CHAPTER 1
INTRODUCTION

Increased interest in psychological assessment in the last few years, particularly in the use of projective techniques, can be traced to three main sources. First, there is a demand for the kind of information that these tests provide. For example, psychodynamic processes can be assessed, as can the apparent presence or absence of neurotic or psychotic processes, contact with reality, general life style, and so on. Second is the continued demonstration that these tests do work despite difficulties in "validation studies." The development of useful, specific scales with demonstrated validity such as the *Rorschach Prognostic Rating Scale* (Klopfer, Ainsworth, Klopfer, & Holt, 1954), as well as comprehensive studies of anxiety, acting out, and suicide, has obviously reinforced the regard in which psychological assessments are held. Third, a number of new texts have appeared which have rekindled interest in projective tests. Among them are Exner's (1974, 1978) two volumes on the Rorschach, Hutt's (1977) volume on the Bender-Gestalt, DeCato and Wicks' (1976) case studies with the Bender-Gestalt, and Wolman's (1978) treatise on clinical diagnosis. As long as psychological tests yield information useful for clinical understanding and decision making, they will be used.

At least once in each generation, a "new" therapeutic approach is heralded by overzealous practitioners and theorists as a panacea for psychological disturbances, and psychological assessment is declared unnecessary. In the 1940s Carl Rogers' nondirective or client-centered therapy was accompanied by predictions of the end of the need for test evaluations. The counselor reflected feelings, the client got better, tests were not needed. Twenty years later, more or less, an essentially comparable pronouncement accompanied the advent of the new "behavior therapies." Unwanted behavior was described, a program was written and implemented, the patient got better, and tests were again considered unnecessary. Between these events, some phenomenological therapists argued against the need for psychological test evaluations. Assessment should have been overkilled and yet the necessity for psychological assessments via tests persists.

The continued importance of psychological assessment has also been documented in a report by Fein (1979). She found that 37% of the working time of psychologists was used for testing in inpatient settings, and further noted that "psychological testing is currently viewed as a significant dimension of mental health services and is applied as diagnostic needs indicate" (p. 874). These assessments were used for estimating potentials, identifying organicity, and pointing to appropriate intervention or therapeutic programs.

Assessments are meaningful and valid to the extent that they contribute positively to the therapeutic program. Fein reasoned that "If we can gain some understandings from projective test data as to why a given patient manifests a maladaptive condition and if from that knowledge we can direct the therapeutic process toward alleviation of the factors that sustain the maladaptive behaviors, then . . . such testing . . . is fully warranted" (p. 874). Her data, collected at the end of one year of therapy and including patients' answers to questions concerning their perception of progress in therapy, indicated that test interpretations had enabled the therapist to get behind resistances faster than was the case when psychological assessments had not guided the therapeutic program. Fein predicted a resurgence of requests for psychological assessments.

Functions of Psychological Assessment

Psychological test data serve many purposes. These range from personnel selection, for which this volume may be minimally helpful (as in signs of ego strength evaluations or evaluations of executives for indices of incipent maladjusting tendencies), to helping subjects, clients, or patients better understand themselves.

Other uses include evaluations in counseling and psychotherapy. An initial need for such help may be assessed as well as the presence or absence of improvement or a need for continuation in therapy. Judicial decisions and commitments related to conditions of sanity, insanity, or mental retardation are often supported by information that reflects the relative objectivity of psychological test findings. Also pertinent here is the use of tests to contribute to decisions regarding qualifications for special help and training in special education and rehabilitation programs. While it is possible to make these kinds of decisions on the basis of interview impressions, recall of past events, or preliminary information from the patient's past medical history, most professionals, both in and out of psychology, feel more comfortable when relatively objective test data contribute to the decision-making process.

Rabin and Hayes (1978) have reviewed Thorne's description of the functions of diagnosis. These functions include:

1. Demonstrating etiological factors, however conceptualized, and especially differentiating between functional and organic disorders.

2. Estimating the degree or intensity of a symptom or disability.
3. Providing a rational basis for a preferable therapeutic approach or approaches.
4. Providing a rational basis for discussing the individual's problems.
5. Determining the prognosis or probable course of the condition.

As the primary function of science is understanding, the primary function of psychological assessment is to understand individuals, how they developed the conditions in which we find them, and what to do about it, if anything. One of the aims of this volume is to contribute toward this goal.

The Appropriate Use of Diagnostic Signs

To arrive successfully at valid interpretive hypotheses and diagnostic impressions, the importance of global analyses cannot be overemphasized. Teaching students to utilize a molar approach is most difficult but must be considered of great importance (Hammer, 1978). The user of this handbook should keep in mind that one cannot develop a valid verbal personality portrait from a mere conglomeration of test signs. Nor will counting signs lead to appropriate diagnostic conclusions. For one cogent impeding factor, the raw number of test signs associated with each symptom or syndrome varies. There are, for example, more than twice as many signs of anxiety contained here as there are signs of repressive-hysterical conditions. Thus, other things being equal, which they aren't, any test battery may be expected to contain more than twice as many indices of anxiety. Even the percentage of signs of a particular condition is not an effective index, for this ignores the qualitative distinction between strong and weak signs which must also enter into the evaluation.

Most students of psychology would feel that one solitary diagnostic sign should not determine a diagnosis. Some are not so clear on the point that five signs of anxiety, for example, do not necessarily make a diagnosis of anxiety. Only a comprehensive qualitative and quantitative evaluation of all pertinent test findings, behavioral observations, and other relevant data can result in valid assessing (Ogdon, 1975). Of course, a test is only a sample of behavior no matter how objective, reliable, valid, and otherwise adequate it may be. "The wise and careful clinician will extend his [or her] analysis based on other test findings, the history of the individual, and other pertinent information such as physical and medical findings" (Hutt, 1978, p. 346). The interpretive process should *begin*, then, with a review and overview of all the relevant data (Exner & Clark, 1978).

Directions for Research

As the use of all the relevant data in psychological assessment continues, there is a continued need for research in this area. It is hoped that as the reader proceeds through the text, areas of needed research will become clear. An obvious area in which a significant research breakthrough seems imminent is in the study of contraindications. This would appear to be a neglected area in which subsequent research should soon make a significant contribution to the study of differential diagnosis.

Another neglected avenue of potentially significant research may lie in the study of the absence of particular test signs in protocols of individuals with a given condition or syndrome. It certainly could be helpful to know where schizophrenics, for instance, do *not* respond to a particular test in a particular way.

Normality is more than the absence of maladjustment. There is considerable room for the development of a positive description of normal, satisfactorily adjusting individuals utilizing test signs. Comprehensive research in the area remains to be undertaken.

The approach of objectively establishing the *relative validity* of specific test signs has yet to be systematically explored. Most test signs are associated with more than one condition or symptom. It would be very helpful to have probability figures associated with each sign-symptom relationship. One clinician's appraisal of the relative validity of relationships between test signs and behavioral referents is available (Ogdon, 1975). Access to more than one such appraisal would certainly be preferable.

As noted in Ogdon (1975), "Eventually, reliable test signs, simple or complex, will become specifically associated, at known levels of probability, with different aspects of normal and abnormal behavior. We now have a large body of knowledge concerning the responses associated with normals, neurotics, psychotics, specific types of neuroses and psychoses, behavioral disorders, life styles, symptoms, ego defenses, personality traits, and so forth. It is time to turn to the search for those signs which have a high probability of being associated with some particular behavioral referent and a low probability of being associated with any other behavioral referent" (p. 5).

CHAPTER 2
NORMALITY AND MINOR PERSONALITY ANOMALIES
NORMALITY

Behavior of Normal People

Describing the behavioral characteristics of normal individuals is perhaps more difficult than providing comparable information for any other section of this handbook. It is virtually impossible to develop a finite list of behaviors which is definitive of a normal person in the manner of describing psychotic behavior or defining a phobia. Adding to the problem is an awareness that normality is a matter of degree, though this may also be said for some of the syndromes described herein. Generally speaking, two classes of people find their way into the offices of psychologists or psychiatrists. First, there are those individuals who find themselves so dissatisfied with their lot in life, with their anxiety, depression, phobias, etc., that they seek professional help to enable them to "get more out of life." The other group may or may not be satisfied with the way their lives are going, but their behavior is so disquieting to the people around them that their relatives, friends, or others force them, sometimes literally, into a setting where they will get help to make their behavior more acceptable. These two broad classes of people are not considered normal. While it is probably true that the absence of any particular behavior or behaviors does not mean a person is normal, normal individuals are largely free from symptoms of neurosis and psychosis. We may use this approach, then, to define normality as the extent to which individuals' behavior is satisfying both to themselves and to the group in which they live. This gives recognition to the fact that there are dimensions of normality—that one may be more or less normal and that this varies at different times and in different places. The complexity of completely describing or defining normality remains a philosophical conundrum.

Granting that there is no altogether acceptable consensus regarding the characteristics of normality, many authors on the subject have recognized that the following qualities are among those typically found in normal individuals. Our thinking here was influenced most by Lehner and Kube (1955).

First, there is a balance between a sense of individuality or independence and a sense of belongingness, of being a part of a group of individuals with whom we interact, for whom we provide goods or services in the broadest sense, and from whom we receive goods or services. Included here is recognition that we are not all alike, but also that we should not all be alike. A part of this is acceptance of our uniqueness as well as a recognition of our human interdependence.

Second, there is a sense of confidence, both in ourselves and in others. This is based on a realistic sense of respect for ourselves and others. Included in this concept is self-acceptance, acceptance not just of our applaudable behavioral tendencies but of our personality liabilities as well.

The dual, intertwined abilities to love and be loved represent additional characteristics of normals, characteristics which most neurotics do not have. To give love to another individual and to be able to accept that individual's love in return are abilities most sensitive to inadequacies in self-respect. A person who lacks self-respect tends to be unable to believe another could love him or her and thus rejects overtures of love from others. On the other hand, only a narcissist can accept another's love and be unable to give love in return. In both instances the deficiency in realistic self-respect and confidence plays a causal role.

The fourth quality is appropriate psychological perspective. Normal people are oriented appropriately as to place, time, and person. More than this, they do not seem to confuse the consequential with the inconsequential. The behavior of normals indicates that they do not overrespond to trivial accomplishments or failures nor do they underrespond to great successes or catastrophes. The concern and responses of normal individuals befit the circumstances. A particular gain or loss, or threatened gain or loss, may have different phenomenal meaning for each of us, but most of us can perceive and differentially respond to winning a door prize at the Saturday club dance and being elected governor of the state, or between the loss of a pet and the loss of a son or daughter.

A sense of flexibility also characterizes normal people. They are capable of modifying their behavior in the pursuit of a goal or of changing the goal itself in the light of current needs and information. Normal individuals are also capable of persevering, but they persevere without blindly perseverating. Changes in attitude and overt behavior accompany perceptual changes of the circumstances and situations in which one finds oneself. Rigidity, for example, leads to abnormal adjusting while flexibility permits normal adjustive behavior.

Finally, there is the ability to enjoy life, the capacity to enjoy oneself, others, and the environment. Every minute of every day is not fun for normal people, but the capacity to enjoy the satisfactions of living is there to balance the frustrations and disappointments. This final characteristic can be summed up as the satisfaction we get from our various roles in life.

Having had the temerity to attempt to describe normal behavior, a final word is imperative. Normality is neither statistical nor ethical perfection. Allport (1937) observed that it is *usual* for individuals to have some noxious trends in their natures, some pathology of tissues or organs, some nervousness, and so forth. In short, most of us are normal, none of us is perfect.

Test Indices

Wechsler Signs

1. **Unusually high Arithmetic score** (Bradway & Benson, 1955).
2. **Unusually high Comprehension score** (Fisher & Sunukjian, 1950; Glasser & Zimmerman, 1967; Gurvitz, 1951; Krippner, 1964; Mayman, Schafer, & Rapaport, 1951; Rapaport, Gill, & Schafer, 1945; Schafer, 1948; Wechsler, 1958).
3. **Unusually high Picture Arrangement score** (Blatt & Quinlan, 1967; Glasser & Zimmerman, 1967; Rapaport et al., 1945).

Rorschach Signs

1. **Average or better than average quality M responses given** (Adams, Cooper, & Carrera, 1963; Alcock, 1963; Hersch, 1962; Kagan, 1960; Klopfer et al., 1954; Klopfer & Davidson, 1962; Lerner & Shanan, 1972; Meyer, 1961; Phillips & Smith, 1953).
2. **Average or greater number of M responses given** (Adams et al., 1963; Allen, 1954, 1958; Barrell, 1953; Dana, 1968; Goldfried, Stricker, & Weiner, 1971; Klopfer & Davidson, 1962; Levine, Glass, & Meltzoff, 1957; Levitt & Truumaa, 1972; Nickerson, 1969; Phillips & Smith, 1953; Piotrowski, 1957, 1960; Schumer cited in Sarason, 1954; Singer, 1955, 1960; Singer & Sugarman, 1955; Singer, Wilensky, & McCraven, 1956; Spivack, Levine, & Sprigle, 1959; Wagner, 1971).
3. **M responses given with H content** (Allen, 1954; Klopfer et al., 1954; Mukerji, 1969; Phillips & Smith, 1953; Piotrowski, 1957).
4. **$M = FM$ where $M = 3$ or more** (Klopfer & Davidson, 1962).
5. **Average number of FM given** (Ames, Learned, Metraux, & Walker, 1952; Ames, Metraux, Rodell, & Walker, 1974; Ames, Metraux, & Walker, 1959, 1971; Klopfer et al., 1954; Piotrowski, 1957).
6. **Average quality FM responses given** (Klopfer et al., 1954).

7. **Average number of FC responses given** (Ames et al., 1952, 1959, 1971, 1974; Beck, 1945; Klopfer & Davidson, 1962; Rorschach, 1921/1951; Schachtel, 1966; Shapiro, 1960).
8. **FC responses in greater number than $CF + C$** (Exner, 1974; Klopfer & Davidson, 1962; Meyer, 1961; Piotrowski, 1957; Vinson, 1960).
9. **Average number of Fc responses given** (Adams et al., 1963; Bochner & Halpern, 1945; Hertz, 1948, 1949; Klopfer & Davidson, 1962; Mons, 1950; Munroe, 1950; Phillips & Smith, 1953; Rapaport, Gill, & Schafer, 1946).
10. **Average or better than average quality F responses given** (Beck, 1960; Klopfer & Davidson, 1962; Korchin, 1960).

Projective Drawing Signs

Detailing

Normal individuals will include essential details in their drawings plus a limited number of details which are not essential and perhaps a few which are constructive but irrelevant. Buck (1948) has described essential details for drawings of persons, trees, and houses. The essential details in a drawing of a person include a head, trunk, two legs and two arms, two eyes, a nose and mouth, and two ears unless an omission is accounted for by the mode of presentation, view, or an appropriate verbal explanation.

The essential details of a House drawing include "at least one door (unless the side of the house only is presented), one window, one wall, and a roof, and unless it is identified as a tropical dwelling, a chimney" (Buck, 1948, p. 50). A Tree drawing of a normal individual should include a trunk and at least one branch (Buck, 1948).

Placement

Central placement is most common for all projective drawings for individuals at all ages (Lakin, 1956; Urban, 1963; Wolff, 1946).

Size

The average height of a human figure drawing on an 8″ by 11½″ sheet of paper is about seven inches (Urban, 1963). Deviations in size must be considered relative to the size of the paper on which the individual draws.

Tree Drawings

1. **Flexibly organized, appropriately formed branches on Tree drawings suggest normal flexibility** (Aronoff, 1972; Buck, 1948, 1964, 1966; Hammer, 1958; Jolles, 1971; Koch, 1952).

2. **Two-dimensional branch systems which are partially drawn with foliage implied by shading or hatching suggests normality** (Jolles, 1971).

Bender-Gestalt Signs
1. **Approximately accurate size of the stimulus figures reproduced in a logical, orderly arrangement suggests normality in persons of all ages** (Byrd, 1956; Clawson, 1959, 1962; Halpern, 1951; Haworth & Rabin, 1960; Hutt, 1953; Hutt & Briskin, 1960).

PSYCHOLOGICAL DEFENSES AND MECHANISMS

A psychological defense is defined as "a mental attribute or mechanism or dynamism, which serves to protect the person against danger arising from his [or her] impulses or affects" (Hinsie & Campbell, 1970). Strictly speaking, this phenomenon refers to unconscious activities. More than a dozen defense mechanisms have been described in the psychological literature (English & English, 1958; Hinsie & Campbell, 1970; Laughlin, 1979; Symonds, 1946). Most of these defenses, including some major ones, have few unequivocal test sign referents. A survey of the literature has turned up a sufficient number of psychological test indices of certain defense mechanisms to warrant their inclusion in this volume. Repression, regression, fantasy, and projection are reviewed. Rationalization and intellectualization are considered together, as are compensation, overcompensation, and reaction formation which are also considered as a related group of defenses.

An attempt will be made to provide examples of behavioral manifestations of psychological defenses. This challenge may not always be well met. There are two basic reasons for this. Since we are dealing with unconscious cognitive processes, it is not altogether realistic to expect this covert behavior to be unequivocally reflected in overt acts. Each of us realizes that there are differences between what we think and what we say, just as there are disparities between what we say and what we do. There are comparable differences between our unconscious and conscious motives. To further confound the attempt to give behavioral examples of defenses in operation is the observation that our defenses tend to act in concert, not one at a time. Thus, an overt defensive act may result from contemporaneous actions of several defensive processes. A person may be repressing, rationalizing, and projecting more or less simultaneously. Behavioral examples of these dynamisms of adjusting cited in this chapter have not altogether adequately circumvented these difficulties.

REPRESSION

Repression refers to the active process of excluding from consciousness unacceptable or ego-alien thoughts, feelings, wishes, impulses, or other related phenomena. Repressive forces may either prevent unwanted information from entering one's memory or eliminate such information after it has been recognized or perceived by the individual. In the latter case we have what has been considered *motivated forgetting*. Since this term, as with all defense mechanisms, refers to ideational rather than motoric phenomena, manifestations are most often noted in the speech or anamnestic reports of individuals. These verbalizations become the behavioral manifestations of this defense.

Behavioral Manifestations

Behavioral manifestations of repression include the following:
1. The differential forgetting of unpleasant and painful memories as compared to pleasant memories that are typically reported. The "good old days" phenomenon reflects repression. Nietzsche's (cited in Laughlin, 1979) observation to the effect that "My memory tells me I did it while my pride says I could not have done it, and in the end my memory yields" is an example.
2. Many slips of the tongue may reveal bonafide repressed feelings rather than that which we intended to say.
3. The cognitive dissonance of incompatible ideas or values which may be expressed by individuals has been cited as an example of repression in action, for it is the force of repression that prevents us from recognizing our logical inconsistencies.

Test Indices

Wechsler Signs
1. **Unusually low Information score** (Allison, Blatt, & Zimet, 1968; Blatt & Allison, 1968; Holt, 1968; Mayman et al., 1951; Pope & Scott, 1967; Rapaport et al., 1945; Schafer, 1948).
2. **Information score significantly below the Comprehension score** (Allison et al., 1968; Blatt & Allison, 1968; Holt, 1968).
3. **Unusually low Block Design score** (Glasser & Zimmerman, 1967).

Rorschach Signs
1. **F% greater than 50** (Allen, 1958; Allison et al., 1968; Ames et al., 1952, 1974; Beck, 1960; Bochner & Halpern, 1945; Consalvi & Canter,

1957; Halpern, 1953; Hertz, 1948, 1949; Hertz & Paolino, 1960; Klopfer et al., 1954; Korchin, 1960; McCue, Rothenberg, Allen, & Jennings, 1963; Mons, 1950; Murstein, 1958; Piotrowski, 1957; Rossi & Neuman, 1961; Sarason, 1954; Schachtel, 1966; Schafer, 1954; Schwartz & Kates, 1957; Siegal, Rosen, & Ehrenreich, 1962; Singer, 1960).

2. *F* greater than three times *FC* + *CF* + *C* (Klopfer et al., 1954; Schafer, 1954).

3. *F* greater than three times (*M* + *FM*) (Klopfer et al., 1954).

4. **A subnormal number of *M* responses** (Affleck & Mednick, 1959; Klopfer et al., 1954; Levine & Spivack, 1964; Phillips & Smith, 1953; Piotrowski, 1957).

5. *M* **greater than** *FM* **with** *FM* **equal to one or zero** (Klopfer & Davidson, 1962; Rosenzweig & Kogan, 1949).

6. *M* **responses with** *A* **content** (Beck, 1945, 1951).

7. *FC* + *CF* + *C* **approximately zero** (Allen, 1954; Exner, 1974; Hertz, 1965; Klopfer et al., 1954; Palmer, 1970; Phillips & Smith, 1953).

8. *FK* + *Fc* **less than 25% of** *F* (Klopfer & Davidson, 1962).

9. **A subnormal number of** *Fc* **responses** (Adams et al., 1963; Klopfer & Davidson, 1962).

10. **A subnormal number of** *W* **responses** (Schafer, 1954).

11. **Bony or hard Anatomy responses emphasized** (Levitt & Truumaa, 1972; Phillips & Smith, 1953; Rapaport et al., 1946).

12. **A subnormal number of content categories used** (Allen, 1958; Allison et al., 1968; Beck, 1945; Hertz, 1948, 1949; Munroe, 1945; Piotrowski, 1969; Schachtel, 1966).

13. **A subnormal number of responses** (Allen, 1954; Auerbach & Spielberger, 1972; Beck, 1960, 1968; Bochner & Halpern, 1945; Schachtel, 1966).

14. **Vague and unelaborated language used** (Levine & Spivack, 1964; Pope & Scott, 1967).

15. *F* **greater than 3 times** (*M* + *FM* + *FC* + *CF* + *C* + *Fc*) (Klopfer et al., 1954).

16. **A subnormal number of** *FM* (Klopfer & Davidson, 1962; Levine & Spivack, 1964; Rosenzweig & Kogan, 1949).

17. **Subnormal number of inanimate movement responses** (Adams et al., 1963; Allen, 1954; Ames et al., 1952; Klopfer et al., 1954; Piotrowski, 1957).

18. *M* + *FM* **equal to or less than one** (Klopfer & Davidson, 1962; Levine & Spivack, 1964).

19. **Greater than normal number of animal content** (Beck, 1960; Schafer, 1954).

Projective Drawing and Bender-Gestalt Signs

1. **Extreme bilateral symmetry in drawings** (Hammer, 1958; Machover, 1949, 1951; Urban, 1963).

2. **Tree drawn leaning to the right** (Buck, 1948; Jolles, 1971).

3. **Trunk of a Tree drawing is narrower at the base than elsewhere** (Koch, 1952).

4. **Bender reproductions manifest sequential reduction in size** (Hutt & Briskin, 1960).

5. **Crowded, compressed, or cohesive arrangements of Bender figures** (Brown, 1965; Clawson, 1959, 1962; Haworth & Rabin, 1960; Hutt, 1953; Hutt & Briskin, 1960; Woltmann, 1950).

6. **The reproduction of Bender's Figure 6 leaves a majority of the upright line above the crossing point** (Lerner, 1972; Weissman & Roth, 1965).

7. **Legs of figure drawing are pressed closely together, especially if the figure is small** (Machover, 1949; Schildkrout, Shenker, & Sonnenblick, 1972; Urban, 1963).

8. **Figure drawing is overclothed** (Gurvitz, 1951).

REGRESSION

In regression we see an unconscious surrendering, in the face of frustration, of more mature or more recently acquired behavior for behavior which is less mature or more remotely learned. It has been considered a form of "psychological retreat" (Laughlin, 1979), by means of which the individual aims to return to an earlier, more satisfying condition. Regression has been defined psychiatrically as "the act of returning to some earlier level of adaptation" (Hinsie & Campbell, 1970).

Three forms of regression have been distinguished in the psychological literature. Age regression coincides most closely with the psychiatric definition. Such behavior is a reversion to a mode or pattern of responding that is characteristic of an individual at an earlier level of development. Encountering frustration or conflict, an adult who acts like an adolescent or child, an adolescent behaving like a child or infant, or a child acting like an infant may depict this form of regression.

Primitivation suggests a second type of regressive behavior (English & English, 1958; Symonds, 1946). More adequate means of adjusting may be replaced by behavior that is, in a sense, more natural or primitive when a profoundly frustrating or threatening circumstance prevails. The well-studied human stampede at the Coconut Grove fire or resorting to cannibalism when confronting a threat to survival may serve as examples of primitivation. These acts, obviously, probably have not occurred earlier in the individual's life, but rather suggest regression to an archaic level. Though less shocking than these examples, Hinsie and Campbell

(1970) suggest that fainting exemplifies "the most primitive response to a trauma."

Instrumental act regression, the third variation on regression, refers specifically to an experimental psychological phenomenon. An animal, usually an infrahuman mammal, may be taught to make a specific response to avoid a noxious stimulus. Then it is retrained to make a new response to avoid the same unpleasant experience. If the animal is subsequently frustrated in its attempt to make the new response, it may revert (regress) to the old response in an attempt to avoid the noxious situation.

Typically, clinical psychologists are concerned with individuals who engage in behavior that is immature or act in a manner less mature than is appropriate for the person's chronological age or level of development. This is regression in its general state.

Behavioral Manifestations

Behavioral manifestations of regression in adults include crying or pouting, temper tantrums or negativistic behavior, baby talk, increased oral activity, loss of continence, excessive sleep, and stampeding.

Test Indices

Rorschach Signs

1. **M responses of poor quality, M-** (Beck, 1945, 1951, 1960; Klopfer et al., 1954; Mayman, 1977).
2. **M responses with Dd locations and Hd content** (Beck, 1960).
3. **M responses with A content** (Beck, 1945, 1960; Phillips & Smith, 1953).
4. **M responses with Hd content** (Beck, 1960).
5. **DW responses noted** (Dudek, 1972).
6. **An abnormally erratic quality of form level** (Mayman, 1970).
7. **Fabulized combinations with content part one thing, part another** (Carlson, Quinlan, Tucker, & Harrow, 1973; Friedman, 1952, 1953; Goldfried et al., 1971).
8. **FM in greater than average number** (Allen, 1954, 1958; Bochner & Halpern, 1945; Hertz, 1960; Kahn & Giffen, 1960; Klopfer & Davidson, 1962; Mons, 1950; Munroe, 1945; Phillips & Smith, 1953; Piotrowski, 1937a; Rosenzweig & Kogan, 1949; Wagner, 1971).
9. **Cn responses present** (Dudek, 1972).

Projective Drawing Signs

Graphological and General Indices

1. **Upper left-hand corner placement** (Barnouw, 1969; Buck, 1948, 1964, 1969; Jolles, 1971; Weider & Noller, 1953).

2. **Very small drawings** (Hammer, 1968; Machover, 1949; Meyer, Brown, & Levine, 1955; Urban, 1963).
3. **Omission of essential details** (Buck, 1948; Deabler, 1969; Kahn & Giffen, 1960; Ries, Johnson, Armstrong, & Holmes, 1966; Swensen, 1968).

Draw-A-Person/Human Figure Drawing Indices

1. **Drawing appears younger than the subject's age, especially if same sex drawing is a child** (Machover, 1949; McElhaney, 1969; Meyer et al., 1955; Urban, 1963).
2. **Minimal sex differences noted between drawings of a male and female** (Modell, 1951).
3. **Head drawn abnormally large** (Goodman & Kotkov, 1953; Machover, 1949, 1951).
4. **Profile drawn of head with the body in a front view** (Machover, 1949; Modell, 1951).
5. **Small circles used for eyes, especially when they are also used for the nose, mouth, and buttons** (Machover, 1949; Urban, 1963).
6. **Mouth emphasized** (Gurvitz, 1951; Jolles, 1971; Machover, 1949, 1951; Urban, 1963).
7. **Protruding lips drawn** (Meyer et al., 1955).
8. **Neck omitted from the drawing** (Machover, 1949; Mundy, 1972).
9. **The upper part of two parallel unbroken lines from head to feet serves as the trunk** (Machover, 1949).
10. **Rounded trunks drawn** (Gurvitz, 1951; Levy, 1950; Machover, 1949).
11. **A mechanical horizontal extension of the arms drawn at right angles to the body** (Machover, 1949).
12. **Mitten-type hands drawn that obscure the fingers** (McElhaney, 1969).
13. **Long, especially very long fingers drawn** (Machover, 1949; Urban, 1963).
14. **Fingers drawn without hands** (Machover, 1949; Shneidman, 1958).
15. **Petal or grape-like fingers drawn short and rounded** (Buck, 1964; Gurvitz, 1951; Hammer, 1958; Machover, 1949; Schildkrout et al., 1972).
16. **Buttons emphasized, especially when drawn mechanically down the middle of the drawing** (Buck, 1964; Jolles, 1971; Machover, 1949; Michal-Smith & Morgenstern, 1969; Urban, 1963; Wolk, 1969).
17. **A stick figure is drawn** (Reynolds, 1978).

H-T-P House Drawing Indices

1. **An anthropomorphic House drawn** (Meyer et al., 1955).

2. **A very small House drawn** (Buck, 1964).
3. **A double perspective drawn with narrow end walls** (Jolles, 1971).
4. **Very few windows drawn** (Meyer et al., 1955).
5. **An angled chimney drawn** (Buck, 1964; Jolles, 1971).
6. **Tulip or daisy-like flowers spontaneously added to the House drawing** (Buck, 1948, 1964, 1966; Hammer, 1954c; Jolles, 1971).

Tree Drawing Indices
1. **Trunks drawn with thickening and/or constrictions** (Koch, 1952).
2. **Long trunk drawn with a small crown** (Koch, 1952).
3. **A branch drawn low on the trunk** (Koch, 1952).
4. **The Tree drawn as a sapling** (Meyer et al., 1955).
5. **The Tree drawn as a fruit tree** (Fukada, 1969).
6. **Animals drawn peeking from a hole in the trunk** (Jolles, 1971).

Bender-Gestalt Signs
1. **Concreteness, giving Bender figures specific interpretive meanings** (Halpern, 1951).
2. **Dots changed to circles** (Brown, 1965; Weissman & Roth, 1965).
3. **Fragmentation in reproductions** (Guertin, 1954a; Halpern, 1951; Hutt, 1977; Hutt & Briskin, 1960).
4. **Simplification, primitivation, or condensation of the figures** (Bender, 1938; Gilbert, 1969; Goldberg, 1956-57; Guertin, 1952; Halpern, 1951; Hutt, 1953, 1968; Hutt & Gibby, 1970; Woltmann, 1950).
5. **Spontaneous elaborations, embellishments, and doodling added to the reproductions** (Hutt, 1953; Story, 1960).
6. **On Figure 1, letters or numbers used instead of dots** (Brown, 1965).
7. **On Figure 3, reducing the number of dots or reducing the number of component parts; this is a form of simplification** (Hutt & Briskin, 1960).
8. **On Figure 3, using circles for dots** (Brown, 1965).
9. **An orderly sequence begun but final figures crammed in at the bottom or scattered suggests rapid regression under stress** (Hutt, 1953; Hutt & Briskin, 1960).
10. **Dashes are substituted for dots** (Hutt, 1977).

Contraindication

1. **Bender Design 3 is well reproduced** (Weissman & Roth, 1965).

COMPENSATION, OVERCOMPENSATION, AND REACTION FORMATION

Compensation can be defined as a process, outside of conscious awareness, by which an individual attempts to overcome or make up for a real or imagined defect or shortcoming through the development or exaggeration of a real or imagined positive characteristic, asset, or talent. When the perceived defect or shortcoming causes an excessive feeling of inferiority and the striving is exaggerated to a deleterious degree, there is *overcompensation*. Compensation appears as a broad, general principle of adjusting which, by definition, leaves the individual better off as it improves self-concept and the quality of adjusting. Overcompensation is excessive and, again by definition, tends to interfere with adjusting processes, leaving the individual, at best, no better off and perhaps in less satisfactory condition than he or she was prior to overcompensating (cf. English & English, 1958; Hinsie & Campbell, 1970).

Reaction formation can be viewed as a special form, or possibly two special forms, of compensation. It is made up in part of repression because, as with all of these defenses, the process is unconscious. It is related to sublimation as well. Two slightly different processes may be involved here. First, there may be an unconscious development of feelings and/or attributes which are diametrically opposed to the unconscious impulses motivating their development. Second, a reaction formation may involve doing the opposite of an unconscious, ego-alien or socially undesirable act that one is originally inclined to do. Although the two uses of the term are related, the former involves a broader change of attitude. In the latter case, a weakness may actually be turned into a strength. In practice it is often difficult if not impossible to differentiate, in overt behavior, between compensatory activity and either form of reaction formation. Inasmuch as overcompensation employs comparable processes, but simply carries them too far (to a "pathological degree"), and because these processes can rarely be distinguished on psychological tests, these defenses are considered together in this section. When the psychodynamics of given behavior are known, some reaction formations may be detected behaviorally.

Behavioral Manifestations

Behavioral manifestations of compensation, overcompensation, and reaction formation are so diverse that providing exhaustive examples would be redolent of overcompensation. In brief, developing a characteristic, talent, or craft to make up for a poor physique, developing a powerful physique to counterbalance perceived intellectual deficiencies, developing one's intellect to overcome undesirable facial features, becoming protective and concerned because of latent hostility, and becoming quite independent because of strong unconscious dependency needs are all appropriate examples. The last two would particularly fit as examples of reaction formation.

Test Indices

Wechsler and Rorschach Signs

1. **Unusually high Information subtest scores** (Allison et al., 1968; Coleman & Rasof, 1963; Gilbert, 1969; Glasser & Zimmerman, 1967; Gurvitz, 1951; Holt, 1968; Mayman et al., 1951; Pope & Scott, 1967; Rapaport et al., 1945; Wechsler, 1958).
2. **Abnormally large number of *W* responses** (Alcock, 1963; Allen, 1954; Hertz, 1960; Klopfer & Davidson, 1962; Kuhn, 1960; Piotrowski, 1957; Rosenzweig & Kogan, 1959; Schachtel, 1966; Schafer, 1954).
3. ***W-* and *W* vague responses present in significant number** (Allen, 1954; Bochner & Halpern, 1945; Gurvitz, 1951; Klopfer & Davidson, 1962; Sarason, 1954; Schafer, 1954).
4. **Superior quality *FC* responses given to *dr* locations** (Schafer, 1954).
5. ***F%* greater than 50** (Levitt & Truumaa, 1972; Schafer, 1954).
6. **Limbs given as *Hd* content on the Rorschach** (Phillips & Smith, 1953).
7. **A greater than normal number of *Ad* responses** (Allison et al., 1968; Bell, 1948; Klopfer & Davidson, 1962; Thompson, 1965).
8. **Vista responses unusually frequent** (Molish, 1967).
9. **Unusually large number of *Hd* responses given** (Molish, 1967).

Projective Drawing Signs

General and Draw-A-Person/Human Figure Drawing Indices

1. **Placement high on the page** (Buck, 1964; Jolles, 1971; Jolles & Beck, 1953b; Levy, 1950; Machover, 1949).
2. **Very large drawings** (Brick, 1944; Buck, 1964; Goodman & Kotkov, 1953; Hammer, 1958; Machover, 1949; Urban, 1963; Wysocki & Whitney, 1965).
3. **Overemphasis on and strong reinforcement of facial features** (Machover, 1949).
4. **Hair emphasized** (Buck, 1950; Levy, 1950, 1958).

5. **Chin emphasized** (Levy, 1950, 1958; Machover, 1949).
6. **Nose overemphasized or strongly reinforced** (Levy, 1950, 1958; Machover, 1949, 1951).
7. **Abnormally long neck drawn** (DiLeo, 1970; Machover, 1949; Urban, 1963).
8. **Long, strong arms drawn** (Buck, 1948, 1964, 1966; Hammer, 1954c, 1960, 1969b; Jolles, 1971; Koppitz, 1966b, 1966c, 1968; Machover, 1949, 1951, 1958; Urban, 1963).
9. **Large, especially very large hands drawn** (DiLeo, 1973; Jolles, 1971; Levy, 1950, 1958; Machover, 1949; Urban, 1963).
10. **Massive or excessively broad shoulders on drawings by males** (Hammer, 1958, 1969b; Levy, 1950; Machover, 1949).

H-T-P House and Tree Drawing Indices

1. **A very large, page-filling House drawing** (Buck, 1964).
2. **Multiple chimneys drawn** (Hammer, 1954c).
3. **House drawn as seen from above, a bird's eye view** (Buck, 1948, 1964; Hammer, 1954c, 1958; Jolles, 1971; Landisberg, 1969).
4. **Excessive branches drawn on a small trunk** (Buck, 1948; Hammer, 1954c; Jolles, 1971).
5. **Periphery of tree trunk is strongly reinforced** (Jolles, 1971).
6. **Two-dimensional leaves drawn which are too large for the branches** (Jolles, 1971).
7. **Tree drawing placed high on the page** (Levy, 1950).
8. **Tree drawing is enormous** (Buck, 1964).

Bender-Gestalt Signs

1. **Unusually large reproductions** (Clawson, 1962; Hutt, 1953, 1977; Hutt & Briskin, 1960).
2. **Rigidly methodical arrangements** (Halpern, 1951).
3. **Overlapping of rows at the end of Figure 2 so that an arrowhead sort of figure results** (Hammer, 1954b).

FANTASY

Not all professionals are convinced that fantasy is an authentic psychological defense mechanism (cf. English & English, 1958; Hinsie & Campbell, 1970; Laughlin, 1979; Symonds, 1946). Part of this reservation lies in the degree to which this cognitive activity is conscious or unconscious. Fantasy is an escape from reality, frustration, conflict, stress, and boredom through imaginal, autistic in the broader sense, activity. It is a partial, temporary dissociation from reality which has unconscious components. Fantasies vary in their relative amount of satisfaction, constructiveness, or healthfulness, as well as degree of realism and consciousness. They may also provide temporary pleasure or sheer enjoyment (Laughlin, 1979). Whether or not it is a genuine psychological defense, fantasy is closely related to the other defenses and often appears to function as one.

Behavioral Manifestations

Behavioral manifestations of fantasy are almost nonexistent. The pensive quietude and wistful smile or vague grimace which frequently accompany this phenomenon are not likely to qualify as behavioral referents for this complex ideational activity, at least not in the opinion of behavioristically oriented psychologists. Occasionally, subsequent verbal reports may reveal that this dynamism has been operating. Literature references cited below have most often related test signs of fantasy either to a priori deductions from theoretical reference frames or to clinical reports of patients.

Test Indices

Rorschach Signs
1. *M* responses with Animal content (Klopfer et al., 1954; Phillips & Smith, 1953).
2. *FC* responses with aggressive content (Sommer & Sommer, 1958).
3. **Greater than average number of** *M* (Allen, 1958; Allison et al., 1968; Ames et al., 1952, 1971, 1974; Beck, 1944, 1951; Cocking, Dana, & Dana, 1969; Dana, 1968; Furrer, 1960; King, 1958, 1960; Kleinman & Higgins, 1966; Klopfer & Davidson, 1962; Lerner, 1966; Mayman, 1977; McCully, 1961; Page, 1957; Palmer & Lustgarten, 1962; Piotrowski, 1937a, 1957; Rorschach, 1921/1951; Singer, 1960; Singer & Herman, 1954).

Projective Drawing Signs
General and Draw-A-Person/Human Figure Drawing Indices
1. **Upper left-hand corner placement** (Buck, 1948; Goodman & Kotkov, 1953; Jolles, 1971; Levine & Sapolsky, 1969; Urban, 1963).
2. **Placement high on the page** (Buck, 1964; Hammer, 1954c, 1958; Jolles, 1969, 1971; Jolles & Beck, 1953b; Urban, 1963).
3. **Edge or bottom placement** (Jolles, 1952a).
4. **Top of paper prevents completion of drawing** (Jolles, 1971).
5. **An abnormally large head on person drawing** (Buck, 1964; Jolles, 1971; Urban, 1963).

6. **An underclothed or nude figure is drawn** (Hammer, 1968; Holzberg & Wexler, 1950; Machover, 1949; Urban, 1963).

H-T-P House Drawing Indices
1. **Roof emphasized through size or shading** (Buck, 1964; Hammer, 1954c, 1958; Jolles, 1971).
2. **House drawn only as a roof but not as an A-frame dwelling** (Buck, 1964; Hammer, 1954c).
3. **Strong overemphasis of the vertical dimension of the House drawing** (Buck, 1964; Jolles, 1971).

Tree Drawing Indices
1. **Tall branches extending off the top of the page** (Buck, 1948, 1964; Hammer, 1958; Jolles, 1971).
2. **Tall, narrow branches that reach up, not out** (Hammer, 1958).
3. **An enormous Tree drawn** (Buck, 1964).
4. **A cloud-like tree crown drawn** (Koch, 1952).

Bender-Gestalt Signs
1. **Loops substituted for dots on Figure 1** (Lerner, 1972).
2. **The diamond displaced to the left in Figure 8** (Lerner, 1972).

RATIONALIZATION, INTELLECTUALIZATION, AND ISOLATION

Rationalization is defined as unconsciously giving a socially and personally acceptable reason for behavior rather than the real reason. A rationalization thus pleases oneself as well as society by justifying behavior which may be of questionable value and obscuring motives which may be ego alien or antisocial. Of course the process must be unconscious—otherwise it is sheer lying.

Rationalization and intellectualization serve a number of purposes. Primary among them is the maintenance of a satisfying self-concept. Not only are ego-alien motives obscured, but the individual preserves a rational appearance which is generally more acceptable than feeling that one is at the mercy of one's emotions. Other accomplishments of intellectualizing defenses include phenomenal resolution of cognitive dissonance and the reduction of envy or jealousy of other people's success, particularly the success of disliked persons or those considered inferior.

There is also an intellectualizing aspect to the defense called "isolation." Isolation refers to the separating of an idea or object from the emotion or affective charge originally associated with it. Once this separation is accomplished, the dissociated affect is repressed and the now nonemotional idea accounted for rationally. This represents a kind of intellectualizing, partial dissociation which is most frequently seen in obsessive-compulsive conditions (Laughlin, 1979; Symonds, 1946).

Behavioral Manifestations

Behavioral manifestations of rationalization and intellectualizing defenses are difficult to delineate objectively. Verbalized expressions of these defenses include the "sour grapes" response noted when some positive goal object is perceived as unattainable and subsequently is seen as undesirable or inferior, and the "sweet lemon" response noted when a negative goal or undesired circumstance comes to pass and is subsequently perceived as having happened for the best and is actually considered as the desired outcome. Another commonly encountered rationalization is "If I didn't do it, someone else would." Behavioral manifestations of isolation are equally difficult to set forth. Excessive punishment of a child by an adult who has a "very good reason" for being harsh (not being angry), or some instances of platonic love where an illicit sexual motive lies unconsciously behind the "simple but genuine friendship" may be appropriate examples.

Test Indices

Wechsler Signs

1. **Information score is unusually high** (Allison et al., 1968; Coleman & Rasof, 1963; Glasser & Zimmerman, 1967; Gurvitz, 1951; Holt, 1968; Mayman et al., 1951; Pope & Scott, 1967; Rapaport et al., 1945; Wechsler, 1958).
2. **Arithmetic score is unusually high** (Rapaport et al., 1945).
3. **Similarities score is unusually high** (Gurvitz, 1951; Holt, 1968; Rapaport et al., 1945; Schafer, 1948; Wechsler, 1958).
4. **Vocabulary score is unusually high** (Glasser & Zimmerman, 1967; Gurvitz, 1951; Holt, 1968; Mayman et al., 1951; Rapaport et al., 1945).

Rorschach Signs

1. **Greater than normal number of *Fk, kF* and *k* determinants used** (Allen, 1954; Consalvi & Canter, 1957; Gurvitz, 1951; Klopfer & Davidson, 1962; Mons, 1950).
2. **Greater than normal number of Anatomy content used** (Allison et al., 1968; Bochner & Halpern, 1945; Klopfer & Davidson, 1962; Schachtel, 1966).
3. *C* **description determinants used** (Klopfer & Davidson, 1962).
4. *FC + CF + C* **is approximately zero** (Alcock, 1963; Shatin, 1952; Sherman, 1955).

5. **Emphasis on *dr* areas with good form level** (Klopfer & Davidson, 1962).
6. **Greater than average number of *Hd* responses** (Klopfer & Davidson, 1962; Phillips & Smith, 1953).

Projective Drawing and Bender-Gestalt Signs

1. **An elaborated or emphasized belt on the figure drawing** (Machover, 1949).
2. **Placement on the right side of the page** (Buck, 1948, 1950, 1964; Hammer, 1958; Jolles, 1971; Jolles & Beck, 1953a).
3. **Finger joints are detailed** (Levy, 1950, 1958; Machover, 1949; Urban, 1963).
4. **Bilateral symmetry is emphasized** (Hammer, 1958; Machover, 1949, 1951; Urban, 1963).
5. **Reduction in the size or curvature and/or the use of guide lines or dots on Bender Figure 6** (Suczek & Klopfer, 1952; Weissman & Roth, 1965).

PROJECTION

Unconsciously attributing one's own ideas, impulses, etc., to other people describes projection. Projections may also be made onto inanimate objects but this is infrequently a clinical problem. Ideas or motives are not projected randomly; typically it is ego-alien motives which are ascribed to others. Those feelings and tendencies which are uncomplimentary to oneself, immoral, antisocial, or illegal are most likely to be differentially singled out and imputed to others (English & English, 1958; Hinsie & Campbell, 1970; Laughlin, 1979; Symonds, 1946).

If it is true that an honest person trusts everyone, this may serve as an exceptional case in which we see the projection of an ego-syntonic proclivity. Projections of this kind tend to have a reciprocal relationship with introjection or identification processes which operate concurrently. This type of projection does not seem to increase under the influence of frustration as is generally true (Symonds, 1946), and probably is not measured by the test indices enumerated in this section.

Behavioral Manifestations

Behavioral manifestations of projection can be cited. "The person who blames another for his [or her] own mistakes" has been noted as an example of projection (Hinsie & Campbell, 1970). Paranoid normals as well as paranoid patients are suspicious of others as a function of their ego-alien projections. Paranoiacs' tendencies to attribute to individuals in their environment their own hostility and latent homosexual propensities has been mentioned frequently in the literature. Prejudices and scapegoating activities invariably seem to involve significant elements of projection. Of course, normal people are often inclined to blame their athletic equipment for their poor performance.

Test Indices

All Test Signs
1. **Abnormally low Picture Completion subtest score on the Wechsler** (Glasser & Zimmerman, 1967).
2. *M* **determinants with** *Dd* **locations and** *Hd* **content on the Rorschach** (Beck, 1945, 1960; Phillips & Smith, 1953; Piotrowski, 1957).
3. **Excessive detail manifested on the projective drawings** (Hammer, 1965, 1969b).

GENERAL EXCESSIVE DEFENSIVENESS

Test Indices

Projective Drawing Signs
1. **Locks emphasized on the windows of the House drawing** (Buck, 1966).
2. **Rain spouts and gutters emphasized and reinforced on the House drawing** (Buck, 1964, 1966; Hammer, 1954c; Jolles, 1971).
3. **Eaves emphasized on the House drawing** (Buck, 1966; Hammer, 1954c; Mursell, 1969).
4. **Shutters drawn closed on the House drawing** (Jolles, 1971).

MINOR PERSONALITY ANOMALIES

WITHDRAWAL, INHIBITION, AND CONSTRICTION

These three phenomena are considered together for several reasons. Each has frustration as a frequent antecedent condition and tends to result from disturbances in social relations. Individuals who find that dealing with people is disquieting or dissatisfying can attempt to resolve this problem by limiting their contact with others (withdrawal), retreating into themselves and suppressing responses, especially those of a social nature (inhibition), and diminishing their spontaneity and reducing the variability in their thinking and behavior (constriction). All of this effectively minimizes the likelihood of frustration from interpersonal interactions.

Another common factor among these tactics of adjusting is encompassed in the strategy to escape from anxiety. Each in its way helps to accomplish this. Constriction tends to help one avoid new and unusual situations where the probability of frustration is higher, including interpersonal encounters. Inhibition restricts behavior in a way that lowers the likelihood of committing an anxiety-provoking act, while withdrawal makes a constraining contribution similar to both constriction and inhibition. In some respects these three phenomena have a dynamic interaction effect, each in turn affecting and being affected by the other.

Other reasons for considering these traits together lie in the observation that psychological test signs of any one tend to be associated with test signs of the other two (Ogdon, 1975), and the clinical observation that these modes of responding frequently occur together in patients. Symonds (1946) has written that "this withdrawal form of response to frustration is characterized by more or less extreme inhibition" (p. 74).

Behavioral Manifestations

Behavioral manifestations of withdrawal, inhibition, and constriction range from mild shyness and generally following a safe day-to-day routine, as seen in inhibited individuals who are normal, to the coarctated life style of a hermit that may be the quintessential example of this syndrome carried to its extreme (short of escape through psychosis). Note that accentuated withdrawal is itself a behavioral manifestation of other nosological entities (e.g., schizophrenia).

Test Indices

Wechsler Signs
1. **Unusually low Information scores** (Harrower, 1956; Wechsler, 1958).
2. **Digit Span scores significantly above Arithmetic** (Ogdon, 1975).

Rorschach Signs
Determinant Signs
1. **Greater than normal number of** *M* **responses** (Barron, 1955; Bendick & Klopfer, 1964; Bochner & Halpern, 1945; Cooper, 1969; Dana & Cocking, 1968; Exner, 1969b; Furrer, 1960; Goldfried et al., 1971; Kagan, 1960; Klopfer & Davidson, 1962; Kuhn, 1960; Kurz, 1963; Levine & Meltzoff, 1956; Levine et al., 1957; Levine & Spivack, 1962; Mann, 1956; McCully, 1961; Meltzoff & Levine, 1954; Meltzoff & Litwin, 1956; Meltzoff, Singer, & Korchin, 1953; Murstein, 1960; Nickerson, 1969; Palmer & Lustgarten, 1962; Piotrowski, 1960; Piotrowski & Dudek, 1956; Rapaport et al., 1946; Rorschach, 1921/1951; Sarason, 1954; Schafer, 1948; Schumer cited in Sarason, 1954; Singer & Herman, 1954; Singer, Meltzoff, & Goldman, 1952; Singer & Spohn, 1954; Singer et al., 1956; Wagner, 1971).

2. **Subnormal number of *M* responses** (Affleck & Mednick, 1959; Klopfer et al., 1954; Levine & Spivack, 1964; Phillips & Smith, 1953; Piotrowski, 1957).

3. ***M* + *FC* equal to zero** (Allison et al., 1968).

4. **Greater than normal number of achromatic responses** (Bohm, 1960; Halpern, 1953; Klopfer & Davidson, 1962; Mons, 1950; Rapaport et al., 1946; Wagner, 1971).

5. **Achromatic plus surface shading responses greater than twice the number of chromatic responses** (Bohm, 1960; Exner, 1974; Klopfer & Davidson, 1962; Wagner, 1971).

6. **No achromatic responses given** (Phillips & Smith, 1953).

7. ***F* responses greater than three times the number of *M* + *FM* + *FC* + *CF* + *C* + *Fc*** (Klopfer et al., 1954; Korchin & Larson, 1977).

8. ***M* determinants with abstract content** (Phillips & Smith, 1953).

9. **Achromatic responses are greater than twice the number of chromatic responses** (Klopfer et al., 1954).

Other Rorschach Signs

1. **Subnormal number of *W* responses** (Bohm, 1958; Cox & Sarason, 1954; Doris, Sarason, & Berkowitz, 1963; Eichler, 1951; Levitt & Grosz, 1960; Neuringer, 1962; Phillips & Smith, 1953; Rapaport et al., 1946; Riessman & Miller, 1958; Sarason, 1954; Schachtel, 1966; Schafer, 1954; Schwartz & Kates, 1957).

2. **Greater than normal number of *D* locations used** (Beck, 1945, 1960, 1968; Levitt & Truumaa, 1972).

3. ***do* responses present** (Allen, 1954; Allison et al., 1968; Ames et al., 1952; Auerbach & Spielberger, 1972; Beck, 1945; Bochner & Halpern, 1945; Bohm, 1958; Eichler, 1951; Holt, 1968; Piotrowski, 1957; Rapaport et al., 1946; Rorschach, 1921/1951; Sarason, 1954).

4. **A subnormal number, especially a void of *H* content** (Allen, 1954; Allison et al., 1968; Arnaud, 1959; Klopfer et al., 1954; Phillips & Smith, 1953).

5. **(*H*) responses present in significant number** (Allen, 1954; Klopfer & Davidson, 1962; Phillips & Smith, 1953).

6. ***H* + *Hd* equal to zero** (Piotrowski, 1969).

7. **A subnormal number of content categories utilized** (Allen, 1958; Allison et al., 1968; Beck, 1945; Exner, 1974; Hertz, 1948, 1949; Munroe, 1945; Piotrowski, 1969; Schachtel, 1966).

8. **A subnormal number of *O* responses** (Hertz, 1948, 1949).

9. **A subnormal number of responses** (Allen, 1954; Auerbach & Spielberger, 1972; Beck, 1960, 1968; Bochner & Halpern, 1945; Schachtel, 1966).

10. **VIII-IX-X% less than 30** (Klopfer et al., 1954).

11. **Use of black on Cards III and V** (Ames & Gillespie, 1973).

Projective Drawing Signs
Graphological and General Signs

1. **Abnormally heavy pressure** (Deabler, 1969; Hammer, 1969a; Handler & Reyher, 1964, 1965, 1966).

2. **Abnormally small drawings** (Alschuler & Hattwick, 1947; Buck, 1964; DeCato & Wicks, 1976; Gilbert, 1969; Halpern, 1951; Hammer, 1954c, 1958, 1968; Jolles, 1971; Kadis, 1950; Koppitz, 1966c; Levine & Sapolsky, 1969; McHugh, 1966; Precker, 1950; Rosenzweig & Kogan, 1949; Waehner, 1946).

3. **Placement on the right side of the page** (Buck, 1964; Hammer, 1965, 1969b; Jolles, 1971; Wolff, 1946).

4. **Placement in any corner** (Hammer, 1958).

5. **Upper left-hand corner placement** (Buck, 1948; Goodman & Kotkov, 1953; Jolles, 1971; Levine & Sapolsky, 1969; Urban, 1963).

6. **Side edge of paper utilized in drawing** (Jolles, 1971).

7. **Abnormal lack of detail in the drawing** (Buck, 1948, 1964, 1966; Schildkrout et al., 1972).

Draw-A-Person/Human Figure Drawing Signs

1. **Facial features omitted** (Gurvitz, 1951; Hammer, 1954c; McElhaney, 1969).

2. **Facial features abnormally dim, especially if drawing is in profile** (Levy, 1958; Machover, 1949; Urban, 1963).

3. **Back of head depicted in drawing** (Buck, 1966).

4. **Pupils omitted from eyes** (Hammer, 1954c, 1958, 1968; Kahn & Giffen, 1960; Levine & Sapolsky, 1969; Machover, 1949; Schildkrout et al., 1972; Urban, 1963).

5. **Person is drawn in profile** (Buck, 1964; Deabler, 1969; Exner, 1962; Hammer, 1954c; Jolles, 1971; Urban, 1963).

6. **Arms omitted from the drawing** (Buck, 1966; DiLeo, 1973; Gilbert, 1969; Gurvitz, 1951; Halpern, 1965; Hammer, 1954c; Holzberg & Wexler, 1950; Jolles, 1969, 1971; Kahn & Giffen, 1960; Kokonis, 1972; Koppitz, 1966a, 1968; Levy, 1958; Machover, 1949; Mursell, 1969; Urban, 1963; Vane & Eisen, 1962).

7. **Arms drawn stiff at the sides** (Buck, 1964; Hammer, 1954c; Jacks, 1969; Jolles, 1971; Machover, 1949; Schildkrout et al., 1972).

8. **Legs drawn pressed closely together** (Machover, 1949; Schildkrout et al., 1972; Urban, 1963).

9. **Short, especially very short legs drawn** (Buck, 1964; Jolles, 1971; Urban, 1963).

10. **Small, especially tiny feet drawn** (Brown, 1958; Buck, 1964, 1966, 1969; DiLeo, 1973; Jolles, 1971; Machover, 1949; Urban, 1963).

H-T-P House Drawing Signs

1. **House drawing has a very distant appearance** (Buck, 1964; Hammer, 1958; Jolles, 1971).

2. **House drawn as seen from below, a worm's eye view** (Buck, 1948; Jolles, 1971).

3. **Only one side wall drawn for a House drawing** (Buck, 1948, 1964, 1966; Hammer, 1958; Jolles, 1971).

4. **An abnormally small House drawing** (Buck, 1948, 1964; Hammer, 1958).

5. **Rear of House drawn** (Jolles, 1971).

6. **Door the last part of the House drawn** (Buck, 1948, 1966; Jolles, 1971).

7. **An abnormally small door drawn** (Buck, 1948, 1964; Hammer, 1954c, 1958; Jolles, 1971).

8. **Doors omitted from the drawing** (Buck, 1948; Hammer, 1954c; Jolles, 1971).

9. **Doors drawn as heavily hinged or locked** (Buck, 1948, 1964, 1966; Hammer, 1954c, 1958; Jolles, 1971).

10. **Shutters drawn closed** (Jolles, 1971).

11. **Windows omitted from the House drawing** (Buck, 1948; Hammer, 1954c; Jolles, 1971).

12. **Curtained windows drawn** (Buck, 1948, 1964; Hammer, 1954c, 1958; Jolles, 1971).

13. **Steps drawn leading to a blank wall** (Buck, 1948; Hammer, 1954c; Jolles, 1971).

14. **A single line drawn for the roof** (Jolles, 1971).

Tree Drawing Signs

1. **Tree drawing is a dead tree** (Hammer, 1958).

2. **Abnormally small Tree drawing** (Buck, 1948, 1969; Hammer, 1954c; Jolles 1971).

3. **Crown of Tree drawing flattened** (Koch, 1952).

4. **Tree trunk drawn narrower at the base than elsewhere** (Koch, 1952).

5. **Abnormal thickening and/or constrictions of the tree trunk** (Koch, 1952).

Bender-Gestalt Signs

1. **Decreased angulation** (Hutt, 1953; Hutt & Briskin, 1960).

2. **Curvature flattened** (Clawson, 1959; DeCato & Wicks, 1976; Halpern, 1951; Hutt, 1953; Hutt & Briskin, 1960).

3. **Abnormally small reproductions** (Clawson, 1959, 1962; DeCato & Wicks, 1976; Gilbert, 1969; Guertin, 1952, 1955; Halpern, 1951; Haworth & Rabin, 1960; Hutt, 1977; Hutt & Briskin, 1960; Mundy, 1972).

4. **Crowded, compressed, or cohesive arrangements** (Brown, 1965; Clawson, 1959, 1962; DeCato & Wicks, 1976; Guertin, 1955; Haworth & Rabin, 1960; Hutt & Briskin, 1960; Woltmann, 1950).

5. **Figure A placed in upper left-hand corner** (Hutt, 1953).

6. **The diamond displaced to the left in Figure 8** (Lerner, 1972).

7. **Sequential reduction in figure size** (Hutt, 1977).

IMMATURITY-DEPENDENCY

Immaturity designates a condition in which we see modes of behaving and adjusting which are not commensurate with one's chronological age but rather are appropriate for someone younger. Often this reflects a failure to develop such modes. In other instances this may result from regressing from a more mature condition, type of response, or style of life to one that is no longer appropriate. Regression nearly always implies a degree of immaturity, though immaturity does not necessarily point to regression. In either instance we have behavior that would be more apropos at an earlier age or stage of development (English & English, 1958).

Dependency suggests a greater than normal need for nurturing and supportive responses from others. This includes exaggerated needs for mothering, affection, protection, and the like (cf. Hinsie & Campbell, 1970). In a general sense, immaturity and dependency both occur in youngsters and are normal for them. Children are, realistically, dependent upon adults and by adult standards have not developed a mature orientation or perspective.

We arrived at the decision to deal with immaturity and dependency together as a function of the test indices of one overlapping with test indices of the other. Laughlin (1979) reached a comparable decision by way of psychotherapeutic experience. He stated, "In the large group of neurotic reactions we have found it convenient and useful clinically to regard Regression as a dependency-seeking process" (p. 338).

Psychodynamically, this condition is expressed in two ways. Frustration is basic to both. Extreme or chronic frustration may produce a fixation at a developmental level which can result in generalized immaturity. Second, frustration may trigger regressive processes causing a reversion to immature behavior.

Behavioral Manifestations

Behavioral manifestations of immaturity-dependency overlap considerably with those associated with regression. In general, any mode of responding that is characteristic of a significantly younger person exhibits this condition. Additionally, an inability to make decisions (abulia) as well as seeking advice and support from others mark the behavior of immature-dependent individuals.

Test Indices

Rorschach Signs

Determinant Signs

1. **Abnormally high number of *FM* responses** (Alcock, 1963; Allen, 1954, 1958; Bochner & Halpern, 1945; Hertz, 1960b; Kahn & Giffen, 1960; Klopfer & Davidson, 1962; Mons, 1950; Munroe, 1945; Phillips & Smith, 1953; Piotrowski, 1937a; Rosenzweig & Kogan, 1949; Wagner, 1971).
2. ***M* responses with *Hd* content** (Phillips & Smith, 1953; Piotrowski, 1957).
3. ***M* responses with *A* content** (Klopfer et al., 1954; Phillips & Smith, 1953).
4. ***FM* responses with food getting or eating content** (Arnaud, 1959).
5. ***FM* responses with passive gratification, being cared for, etc.** (Arnaud, 1959).
6. **Abnormally large number of *cF* responses** (Klopfer & Davidson, 1962).
7. ***CF* responses unusually large in number** (Klopfer et al., 1954; Mundy, 1972; Piotrowski, 1957; Rorschach, 1921/1951; Schachtel, 1966).
8. ***FM* is much greater than *M*** (Klopfer & Davidson, 1962; Piotrowski, 1957).

Other Rorschach Signs

1. **Greater than normal number of *A* responses** (Alcock, 1963; Ames & Gillespie, 1973; Halpern, 1960; Palmer, 1970; Phillips & Smith, 1953).
2. **Mountain or hilly landscape content** (Phillips & Smith, 1953).
3. **Visceral or soft anatomy content** (Phillips & Smith, 1953).
4. **Smoke content emphasized** (Phillips & Smith, 1953).
5. **Stroking or patting of ink blots noted** (Klopfer et al., 1954; Phillips & Smith, 1953).
6. **Rotating the cards immediately on presentation** (Phillips & Smith, 1953).
7. **A "pile of rocks" or "leaf" response to Card I** (Ames & Gillespie, 1973; Santostefano & Baker, 1972).

8. **A subnormal number, especially a void, of *H* responses** (Fisher, 1962; Klopfer et al., 1954; Palmer, 1970; Rosenzweig & Kogan, 1949).

Projective Drawing Signs

Draw-A-Person/Human Figure Drawing Signs

1. **Very small drawings produced** (Hammer, 1968; Machover, 1949; Meyer et al., 1955; Urban, 1963).
2. **Drawings appearing younger than subject's age** (Machover, 1949; McElhaney, 1969; Meyer et al., 1955; Urban, 1963).
3. **Drawing of the opposite sex looks older than same sex drawing or subject's age** (Hammer, 1954a).
4. **Head drawn abnormally large** (Goodman & Kotkov, 1953; Machover, 1949, 1951).
5. **Small circles drawn for eyes, especially when also used for the nose, mouth, and buttons** (Machover, 1949; Urban, 1963).
6. **Button- or triangle-shaped noses drawn** (Urban, 1963).
7. **Unusually full lips drawn** (Machover, 1949; Urban, 1963).
8. **Concave mouths drawn** (Machover, 1949; Schildkrout et al., 1972; Urban, 1963).
9. **Neck omitted from drawing** (Machover, 1949; Mundy, 1972).
10. **Breasts omitted in females' drawings** (Brown, 1958).
11. **Unusually large breasts drawn by males** (Hammer, 1954c; Jolles, 1971; Levy, 1950, 1958; Machover, 1949, 1951; Urban, 1963).
12. **Buttocks emphasized** (Jolles, 1971; Urban, 1963).
13. **Short and rounded petal or grape-like fingers** (Buck, 1964; Gurvitz, 1951; Hammer, 1958; Machover, 1949; Schildkrout et al., 1972).
14. **Joints emphasized in drawings** (Levy, 1958; Machover, 1949).
15. **Pockets emphasized** (Levy, 1958; Machover, 1949, 1951; Urban, 1963).
16. **Buttons emphasized** (Halpern, 1958; Hammer, 1954c; Jolles, 1971; Levy, 1950, 1958; Machover, 1949, 1951, 1955, 1958; Reynolds, 1978; Schildkrout et al., 1972; Urban, 1963).
17. **A row of irrelevant buttons drawn down the midline of the drawing** (Hammer, 1954c; Machover, 1949, 1955; Schildkrout et al., 1972; Urban, 1963).
18. **Person drawn as a cowboy** (Hammer, 1958).
19. **Ground lines sloping downward on both sides of the figure** (Hammer, 1954c; Jolles, 1971; Mursell, 1969).

20. **Edge placement used** (Hammer, 1958; Reynolds, 1978).

H-T-P House and Tree Drawing Signs
1. **Tulip or daisy-like flowers spontaneously added to House drawing** (Buck, 1948, 1964, 1966; Hammer, 1954c; Jolles, 1971).
2. **Tree drawing is quite small and isolated on a hilltop** (Buck, 1948, 1964, 1966; Jolles, 1971).
3. **Tree is drawn as a sapling** (Buck, 1948; Hammer, 1958).
4. **Christmas tree drawn not during the Christmas season** (Hammer, 1954c).
5. **A fruit tree is drawn** (Fukada, 1969).
6. **A large trunk drawn with a small branch structure** (Jolles, 1971).
7. **Animals drawn peeking from a hole in the trunk** (Jolles, 1971).
8. **A very large door on the House drawing** (Buck, 1964; Hammer, 1954c, 1958; Jolles, 1971).

Bender-Gestalt Signs
1. **Overlapping and crossing difficulty** (Hammer, 1954b; Hutt & Gibby, 1970).
2. **Figure 2 organized by rows rather than by columns** (Bender, 1938; Keller, 1955).
3. **Figure 5 reproduced abnormally large** (Lerner, 1972).
4. **Drawing the diagonal of Figure 5 inward toward the hoop** (Peek, 1953).
5. **Regression including simplification and condensation** (Bender, 1938; Clawson, 1959, 1962; DeCato & Wicks, 1976; Halpern, 1951; Koppitz, 1958).
6. **Difficulty in joining the elements of Figure 4** (DeCato & Wicks, 1976).

Contraindications

1. *M* **determinants with abstract content** (Phillips & Smith, 1953).
2. **"Two kids dancing" response to Rorschach Card I** (Ames & Gillespie, 1973; Santostefano & Baker, 1972).

INSECURITY, INADEQUACY, AND INFERIORITY

Insecurity implies that an individual feels or behaves in ways that suggest an inability or inadequacy to protect oneself from danger. The danger may be physical or it may be psychological such as protecting one's self-concept. A degree of apprehension is suggested. Insecurity has a situational connotation, although some individuals may be more or less chronically insecure. Inadequacy suggests that the person does not feel equal to the challenges being faced. Psychological skills necessary to reduce frustrations are felt to be lacking. Inferiority also suggests subnormal quality or value. As with inadequacy, a condition is suggested that is below par. The term *inferiority* seems to imply a more durable trait.

These characteristics, while differentially definable, are often associated in common parlance with an "inferiority complex" (Webster's New World Dictionary, 1976). One of the links between these traits is aggression. Of course, aggressive treatment may cause this triad of experiences. On the other hand, one's own aggressive behavior frequently reflects feelings of inferiority as aggressive behavior serves both to obscure the ego-alien feelings and to implement the hope of generating a more secure situation (Symonds, 1946). Aggressive responses tend to result from experiences of frustration. Students of psychology are aware that both immediate frustration as well as early or remote frustrating experiences contribute to an individual's level of aggression and insecurity feelings. One of the salient early frustrations may be thwarting of the child's need to be loved. The hostile adult with feelings of inferiority often was the child who was not loved. The feeling of not being loved is, in turn, another common factor binding insecurity, inadequacy, and inferiority. The roots of these feelings, especially of inferiority, seem to lie in early and severe frustration, particularly involving parental love. The common antecedent conditions, the similarity in the feelings they elicit, as well as the common psychological test indices associated with these three unwanted experiences all suggest that they be considered together.

Behavioral Manifestations

Behavioral manifestations of insecurity, inadequacy, and inferiority are numerous, diverse, and disguised through the use of defense mechanisms. Examples fall in the areas of attention-seeking behavior, approval-seeking behavior, exaggerated power- or status-seeking behavior, and manifestations of most defense mechanisms, particularly compensation, reaction formation, and displacement (cf. Laughlin, 1979).

Test Indices

Wechsler Signs
1. **Unusually low Comprehension score** (Glasser & Zimmerman, 1967).
2. **Unusually low Block Design score** (Glasser & Zimmerman, 1967).

Rorschach Signs

Determinant and Location Signs

1. **Flexor *M* responses given** (Allen, 1954; Beck, 1945; Bochner & Halpern, 1945; Levitt, Lubin, & Zuckerman, 1962; Mukerji, 1969; Piotrowski, 1960; Pope & Scott, 1967; Rorschach, 1921/1951; Taulbee, 1961).
2. **Abnormally large number of inanimate movement responses** (Adams et al., 1963; Alcock, 1963; Klopfer et al., 1954, 1956; Klopfer & Davidson, 1962; Phillips & Smith, 1953; Piotrowski, 1960; Schachtel, 1966).
3. **Abnormally large number of *FC* responses** (Klopfer et al., 1954; Schafer, 1954).
4. **Abnormally large number of shading responses** (Hertz, 1948, 1949; Sarason, 1954).
5. **Abnormally large number of *cF* responses** (Beck, 1960; Klopfer & Davidson, 1962; Sarason, 1954).
6. **Abnormally large number of Vista responses** (Allen, 1954; Beck, 1945, 1951, 1960; Beck & Molish, 1967; Beck, Beck, Levitt, & Molish, 1961; Bochner & Halpern, 1945; Hertz, 1948, 1949; Lord, 1950; Molish, 1967).
7. **Abnormally large number of *D* locations used** (Beck, 1945; Klopfer & Davidson, 1962), **or *D, S*** (Fonda, 1977).
8. **Abnormally large number of *d* locations used** (Gurvitz, 1951; Halpern, 1953; Klopfer & Davidson, 1962; Levitt & Truumaa, 1972; Piotrowski, 1957; Schafer, 1954).
9. **Emphasis on *dd* locations** (Klopfer et al., 1954; Schachtel, 1966; Schafer, 1954).
10. **Subnormal or zero number of *S* locations** (Beck, 1945; Fonda, 1960).
11. ***FM* with food getting, eating or passive gratification content** (Arnaud, 1959).

Content Signs

1. **(*H*) responses emphasized** (Arnaud, 1959; Levitt et al., 1962; Phillips & Smith, 1953).
2. **Mouth as an *Hd* content emphasized** (Arnaud, 1959; Levitt et al., 1962; Lindner, 1947; Masling, Rabie, & Blondheim, 1967; Phillips & Smith, 1953; Schafer, 1954; Wiener, 1956).
3. **Abnormally large number of *A* Object content used** (Allen, 1954).
4. **Passive domestic animals and beasts of burden content emphasized** (Bochner & Halpern, 1945; Klopfer & Davidson, 1962; Levitt et al., 1962; Masling et al., 1967).
5. **Breast content emphasized** (Klopfer & Davidson, 1962; Levitt et al., 1962).
6. **Food content emphasized** (Arnaud, 1959; Kagan, 1960; Klopfer & Davidson, 1962; Levitt et al., 1962; Masling et al., 1967; McCully, Glucksman, & Hirsch, 1968; Phillips & Smith, 1953; Schafer, 1954; Thompson, 1965).
7. **Rorschach content of homes emphasized** (Arnaud, 1959; Halpern, 1953; Levitt et al., 1962).
8. **Mountain and hilly landscape content emphasized** (Phillips & Smith, 1953; Piotrowski, 1957).
9. **Nature or water landscape content emphasized** (Phillips & Smith, 1953).
10. **Cliff, canyon, or chasm content used** (Phillips & Smith, 1953).
11. **Island content used** (Phillips & Smith, 1953).
12. **Rock content used** (Halpern, 1953; Potkay, 1971; Rychlak, 1959).
13. **Religion content used** (Levitt et al., 1962; Phillips & Smith, 1953).
14. **Emblem content emphasized** (Lindner, 1947, 1950; Phillips & Smith, 1953).
15. **Plant or botany content emphasized** (Phillips & Smith, 1953).
16. **Blocking or shock to Card IV** (Phillips & Smith, 1953; Piotrowski, 1957).
17. **Bridge content emphasized** (Halpern, 1953; Phillips & Smith, 1953).
18. **Stroking or patting the blots** (Klopfer et al., 1954; Phillips & Smith, 1953).

Projective Drawing Signs

Graphological and General Signs

1. **Abnormally light pressure used** (Buck, 1969; DiLeo, 1970, 1973; Hammer, 1954c, 1968; Jolles, 1971; Kadis, 1950; Machover, 1949; Reynolds, 1978; Rosenzweig & Kogan, 1949; Urban, 1963).
2. **Abnormally variable pressure used** (Machover, 1949; Wolff, 1946).
3. **Interrupted, curvilinear strokes used** (Alschuler & Hattwick, 1947; Hammer, 1958; Precker, 1950; Waehner, 1946).
4. **Sketchy strokes used** (DiLeo, 1973; Halpern, 1951; Hammer, 1954c, 1958; Hutt, 1977; Rosenzweig & Kogan, 1949; Urban, 1963).
5. **Vague lines with vacillating direction and interrupted strokes used** (Jacks, 1969; Levy, 1950, 1958; Hammer, 1954c; Wolff, 1946).
6. **Shading, especially deep shading used** (Buck, 1948).
7. **Abnormally small drawings made** (Alschuler & Hattwick, 1947; Buck, 1948, 1964; DiLeo, 1973; Gray & Pepitone, 1964; Hammer, 1958, 1968; Jacks, 1969; Jolles, 1971; Koppitz, 1966c, 1968;

Lakin, 1956; Lehner & Gunderson, 1948; Levy, 1950, 1958; Ludwig, 1969; Marzolf & Kirchner, 1972; McElhaney, 1969; McHugh, 1966; Michal-Smith & Morgenstern, 1969; Mundy, 1972; Precker, 1950; Urban, 1963).

8. **Very large drawings made** (Brick, 1944; Buck, 1964; Goodman & Kotkov, 1953; Hammer, 1958; Machover, 1949, 1951; Urban, 1963; Wysocki & Whitney, 1965).

9. **Drawing on bottom edge of the paper** (Buck, 1964; DeCato & Wicks, 1976; Hammer, 1954c, 1958; Jolles, 1971; Reynolds, 1978; Schildkrout et al., 1972).

10. **Drawing placed very low on the page** (Buck, 1950, 1964; DiLeo, 1973; Hammer, 1958; Jolles, 1971; Jolles & Beck, 1953b; Mursell, 1969; Urban, 1963).

11. **Drawing placed in a lower corner** (McElhaney, 1969).

12. **Drawing placed in the absolute center of the page** (Buck, 1948, 1950, 1964; Hammer, 1954c; Jolles, 1971; Machover, 1949; Urban, 1963).

13. **Upper left-hand corner placement** (Buck, 1948; Goodman & Kotkov, 1953; Jolles, 1971; Levine & Sapolsky, 1969; Urban, 1963).

14. **Marked disturbance of symmetry** (Hammer, 1958; Mundy, 1972; Wolff, 1946).

15. **Extreme bilateral symmetry in drawing** (Buck, 1966; Hammer, 1954c).

Draw-A-Person/Human Figure Drawing Signs

1. **A stick figure drawn for a person** (Buck, 1948; Hammer, 1954c, 1958; Levy, 1950, 1958; Rosenzweig & Kogan, 1949; Urban, 1963).

2. **Person drawn in a sitting position** (Allen, 1958).

3. **A figure drawn with a wide stance** (Buck, 1964; Hammer, 1969b; Jolles, 1971; Machover, 1949; Urban, 1963).

4. **Figure drawn with a slanting stance as when legs appear to float in space** (Deabler, 1969; Machover, 1949).

5. **Midline stressed through Adam's apple, tie, button, buckle, fly, etc., or line drawn down the middle** (Bodwin & Bruck, 1960; Machover, 1949; Urban, 1963).

6. **Groundline spontaneously added to figure drawing** (Hammer, 1954c; Jacks, 1969).

7. **Head drawn unusually small** (Jolles, 1971; Machover, 1949).

8. **Facial features overemphasized or strongly reinforced** (Machover, 1949).

9. **Nose drawn unusually large or strongly reinforced** (Levy, 1950, 1958; Machover, 1949, 1951).

10. **Chin appears weak** (Urban, 1963).

11. **Chin overemphasized** (Jolles, 1971).

12. **Tiny shoulders drawn** (Buck, 1964; Jolles, 1971; Urban, 1963).

13. **Small, especially very small trunk to person drawing** (Buck, 1964; Jolles, 1971; Urban, 1963).

14. **Thin, especially very thin trunk drawn on one's own sex figure** (Jolles, 1971; Machover, 1949).

15. **Arms omitted from person drawing** (Buck, 1966; DiLeo, 1973; Gilbert, 1969; Gurvitz, 1951; Halpern, 1965; Hammer, 1954c; Holzberg & Wexler, 1950; Jolles, 1969, 1971; Kahn & Giffen, 1960; Kokonis, 1972; Koppitz, 1966a, 1968; Levy, 1958; Machover, 1949; Mursell, 1969; Urban, 1963; Vane & Eisen, 1962).

16. **Frail, flimsy, thin, wasted, shrunken arms drawn** (Brown, 1953; Buck, 1964, 1966; Hammer, 1954c, 1958; Jolles, 1971; Machover, 1949; Mursell, 1969; Reznikoff & Tomblen, 1956; Urban, 1963; Wolk, 1969).

17. **Short, especially very short arms drawn** (Buck, 1964, 1966; Gilbert, 1969; Jolles, 1971; Machover, 1949; Schildkrout et al., 1972; Urban, 1963; Wolk, 1969).

18. **Arms drawn unattached to the trunk** (McElhaney, 1969).

19. **Transparent arms drawn** (Buck, 1969).

20. **Large, especially very large hands drawn** (DiLeo, 1973; Jolles, 1971; Levy, 1950, 1958; Machover, 1949; Urban, 1963).

21. **Hands drawn last** (Buck, 1964; Jolles, 1971; Urban, 1963).

22. **Shaded hands drawn** (Buck, 1964; Jolles, 1971; Koppitz, 1968; Levy, 1950, 1958; Machover, 1949; Urban, 1963).

23. **Fewer than five fingers drawn on the hand** (Schildkrout et al., 1972).

24. **Unusually small hands drawn** (DiLeo, 1973; Hammer, 1954c).

25. **Thin, tiny, shaded, wasted, shrunken legs drawn with a full body** (Hammer, 1958; Machover, 1949; Reznikoff & Tomblen, 1956; Urban, 1963).

26. **Small, especially tiny feet drawn** (Brown, 1958; Buck, 1964, 1966, 1969; DiLeo, 1973; Jolles, 1971; Machover, 1949; Modell & Potter, 1949; Urban, 1963).

27. **Unusually large feet drawn** (Modell & Potter, 1949; Urban, 1963).

28. **Elongated feet drawn** (Buck, 1964, 1966; Hammer, 1953a; Jolles, 1971).

29. **Buttons emphasized or strongly reinforced** (Halpern, 1958; Hammer, 1954c; Jolles, 1971; Levy, 1950, 1958; Machover, 1949, 1951, 1955, 1958; Schildkrout et al., 1972; Urban, 1963).

30. **Clothes drawn too big for the person** (Buck, 1950; Hammer, 1958).

31. **Belt buckles emphasized** (Machover, 1951, 1958).

32. **A male's drawings show a larger, aggressive or muscular female drawing with a wide stance while the male drawing appears relatively emasculated, effeminate, and collapsed** (Levy, 1958; Machover, 1949; McElhaney, 1969; Pollitt, Hirsch, & Money, 1964; Urban, 1963).

33. **A male's drawings depict the male drawing off balance or without hands or feet** (McElhaney, 1969).

H-T-P House Drawing Signs

1. **House drawn as seen from below, a worm's eye view** (Buck, 1964; Hammer, 1958).

2. **A very small House drawing** (Buck, 1948, 1964).

3. **House drawn at the bottom edge of the page** (Buck, 1948, 1964; Jolles, 1971).

4. **Groundline is spontaneously added to House drawing** (Buck, 1964; Hammer, 1954c; Jolles, 1971).

5. **Shrubs spontaneously drawn around the House drawing** (Buck, 1948, 1964, 1966; Hammer, 1954c; Jolles, 1971).

6. **The sun spontaneously included in the House drawing** (Hammer, 1954c; Marzolf & Kirchner, 1972).

7. **Many trees spontaneously drawn around the House drawing** (Levine & Sapolsky, 1969).

8. **A very small door drawn on the House** (Buck, 1964; Hammer, 1958; Jolles, 1971; Mursell, 1969).

9. **A very large door drawn on the House** (Buck, 1964; Hammer, 1954c, 1958; Jolles, 1971).

Tree Drawing Signs

1. **A tiny Tree drawing** (Buck, 1948, 1964; Hammer, 1954c; Jolles, 1971).

2. **The Tree drawn in a depression** (Buck, 1964).

3. **A dead Tree is drawn** (Barnouw, 1969; Hammer, 1958; Jolles, 1969, 1971).

4. **Shaded roots drawn** (Michal-Smith & Morgenstern, 1969).

5. **Roots overemphasized** (Jolles, 1971).

6. **Roots drawn on bottom edge of paper** (Hammer, 1958).

7. **Root structure is poorly organized** (Buck, 1948).

8. **Omission of roots and baseline** (Michal-Smith & Morgenstern, 1969).

9. **A faintly drawn trunk** (Buck, 1964, 1966; Jolles, 1971).

10. **A tiny, thin trunk drawn** (Buck, 1964; Jacks, 1969; Jolles, 1971; Landisberg, 1969).

11. **Broad-based trunks drawn** (Levine & Sapolsky, 1969).

12. **A flattened tree crown drawn** (Koch, 1952).

13. **Tiny branches drawn on large trunks** (Buck, 1969; Hammer, 1954c, 1958; Jacks, 1969; Jolles, 1969).

14. **Broken or cut off branches drawn** (Hammer, 1953a, 1958; Jolles, 1971).

15. **One-dimensional branches drawn that are inadequately related and inadequately joined to the truck** (Hammer, 1954c, 1958; Jolles, 1971; Mursell, 1969).

16. **Two-dimensional leaves drawn that are too large for the branches** (Buck, 1964; Jolles, 1971).

17. **Deep shading on Tree trunk** (Buck, 1948).

Bender-Gestalt Signs

1. **Angulation changes manifested** (Halpern, 1951).

2. **Overlapping and crossing difficulty noted** (Curnutt, 1953; Hammer, 1954b; Hutt & Gibby, 1970; Koppitz, 1958; Story, 1960).

3. **Reduction in size of reproductions** (Clawson, 1962; Gilbert, 1969; Guertin, 1952, 1954b, 1955; Halpern, 1951; Hutt, 1977; Hutt & Briskin, 1960; Mundy, 1972).

4. **A rigidly methodical arrangement** (Halpern, 1951).

5. **On Figure 5, the dots converge** (Hutt, 1977; Lerner, 1972; Weissman & Roth, 1965).

6. **On Figure 5, extending circular dots to complete the circle** (Hutt & Briskin, 1960).

7. **On Figure 5, drawing the diagonal extension inward toward the hoop** (Peek, 1953).

8. **Figure 5 reduced in size and rotated counterclockwise** (DeCato & Wicks, 1976).

9. **Figure 6 drawn with nonintersecting lines** (Hammer, 1954b).

10. **Crowded, compressed, or cohesive arrangement** (Billingslea, 1948; Halpern, 1951; Hutt & Briskin, 1960; Woltmann, 1950).

11. **Reproductions hug the margins** (DeCato & Wicks, 1976; Hutt, 1978).

Contraindication

1. **On projective drawings, using a firm, unhesitating, determined quality of stroke** (Levy, 1950, 1958).

CHAPTER 3
NEUROSES AND NEUROTIC EPIPHENOMENA

Six sections in this chapter deal with neuroses. The first embraces general indices of neurosis, behavioral manifestations and test signs which generally differentiate neurotics from normals, psychotics, and individuals in other major nosological categories. Succeeding sections consider specific aspects or types of neurosis: anxiety, tension, hysterical-repressive neuroses, intellectualizing obsessive-compulsive neuroses, and phobic conditions.

NEUROSES

Neurotics are characterized as disturbed individuals who nevertheless are usually capable of earning a living and maintaining themselves independently outside hospitals or institutions. However, they do tend to be relatively ineffective, inefficient, chronically dissatisfied, easily fatigued people who are tense and rigid in their life style. Anxiety is considered by many to be the nuclear neurotic process. Most neurotic symptoms appear to be aimed at reducing the experience of anxiety, itself the prime neurotic symptom.

In neuroses only a part of the personality is affected. Though neurotic conditions are not healthy or are marked by unsatisfactory adjusting, the cause is not organic, speech is rarely disturbed, they are not accompanied by structural changes, and definitive symptoms of psychosis are absent. Rather, neuroses are considered functional disorders whose etiology is psychological or behavioral (cf. Hinsie & Campbell, 1970; Rycroft, 1973).

Behavioral Manifestations

Behavioral manifestations of neurosis include fear responses, unfounded somatic complaints, inaccurate recollections recounted, numerous dislikes recited, chronic discontent and restlessness verbalized, insatiable needs, an inadequate sex life, sundry preoccupations, and an unrealistic level of aspiration reported. Manifestations of anxiety and tension, recorded elsewhere in this chapter, are also expressions of neuroses, though not exclusively so, as are expressions of guilt and having sinned.

Test Indices

Wechsler Signs
1. **Verbal IQ significantly above Performance IQ, especially for anxiety and tension states, neurasthenia, and obsessive-compulsive conditions** (Gilbert, 1969; Gurvitz, 1951; Mayman et al., 1951; Schafer, 1948; Wechsler, 1958).

2. **Performance IQ significantly above Verbal IQ, particularly for hysterical or cyclothymic types of neurotic conditions** (Allison et al., 1968; Gilbert, 1969; Holt, 1968; Schafer, 1948).
3. **Low Vocabulary scores, especially for neurasthenic conditions** (Holt, 1968; Rapaport et al., 1945).
4. **Low Digit Symbol scores** (Gilbert, 1969; Holland, Levi, & Watson, 1979; Ladd, 1964; Wechsler, 1958).
5. **Low Object Assembly scores** (Holt, 1968).

Rorschach Signs
1. **Subnormal number of *M* responses** (Alcock, 1963; Bohm, 1958; Fisher, 1950; Goldfried et al., 1971; Hertz, 1948, 1949; Kahn & Giffen, 1960; Klopfer & Davidson, 1962; Levine et al., 1957; Miale & Harrower-Erickson, 1940; Munroe, 1945; Nickerson, 1969; Rapaport et al., 1946; Spivack et al., 1959; Vinson, 1960).
2. ***M* + *FM* equals one or zero** (Klopfer et al., 1954).
3. ***FM* greater than 2 *M*** (Alcock, 1963; Goldfried et al., 1971; Hertz, 1948; Klopfer et al., 1954; Miale & Harrower-Erickson, 1940).
4. ***M* with *Hd* emphasized** (Phillips & Smith, 1953).
5. **High frequency of *Fc*** (Bohm, 1960; Raifman, 1957).
6. **Greater than average number of shading responses** (Bohm, 1977; Raifman, 1957).
7. ***F%* greater than 50** (Alcock, 1963; Allison et al., 1968; Beck, 1945; Bochner & Halpern, 1945; Goldfried et al., 1971; Hertz, 1948; Holt, 1968; Kahn & Giffen, 1960; Klopfer et al., 1954; Korchin, 1960; Levi, 1951, 1965; Miale & Harrower-Erickson, 1940; Mundy, 1972; Munroe, 1945; Pope & Scott, 1967; Rapaport et al., 1946; Schafer, 1954).
8. **Unusually high *F+%*** (Berkowitz & Levine, 1953; Levi, 1951; Mayman, 1970; Schafer, 1954).
9. **Subnormal number of *FC*** (Fisher, 1950; Goldfried et al., 1971; Hertz, 1948; Kahn & Giffen, 1960; Kates, 1950; Miale & Harrower-Erickson, 1940; Munroe, 1945; Piotrowski, 1957; Rapaport et al., 1946).
10. **Pure *C* responses present** (Beck, 1945; Fisher, 1950; Goldfried et al., 1971; Phillips & Smith, 1953; Schafer, 1948).
11. **Sum *C* greater than 3** (Haworth, 1962; Hertz, 1948; Murstein, 1960; Rapaport et al., 1946).

12. *FC + CF + C* **is approximately zero** (Alcock, 1963; Shatin, 1952; Sherman, 1955).
13. *CF* **greater than** *FC* (Allison et al., 1968; Beck, 1945; Munroe, 1945).

Location Indices
1. *Dd* **locations emphasized** (Allen, 1954; Allison et al., 1968; Ames et al., 1952, 1974; Beck, 1945; Bochner & Halpern, 1945; Bohm, 1958; Fisher, 1950; Goldfarb, 1943; Goldfried et al., 1971; Gurvitz, 1951; Hertz, 1948; Holt, 1968; Kahn & Giffen, 1960; Klopfer et al., 1954; Levi, 1965; Piotrowski, 1957; Sarason, 1954).
2. **Subnormal number of** *D* (Alcock, 1963; Holt, 1968; Klopfer et al., 1954; Klopfer & Davidson, 1962; Raifman, 1957).

Content Indices
1. **Anatomy responses greater than average in number** (Allen, 1954; Allison et al., 1968; Ames et al., 1952, 1974; Arnaud, 1959; Beck, 1945; Bochner & Halpern, 1945; Bohm, 1958; Brar, 1970; Carnes & Bates, 1971; Goldfried et al., 1971; Halpern, 1953; Kahn & Giffen, 1960; Klopfer & Davidson, 1962; Knopf, 1956, 1965; Levitt & Truumaa, 1972; Lindner, 1946; Mons, 1950; Munroe, 1945; Phillips & Smith, 1953; Piotrowski, 1957; Pope & Scott, 1967; Rapaport et al., 1946; Ross, 1940; Ross & Ross, 1944; Schachtel, 1966; Schafer, 1948; Wagner, 1973).
2. **Animal responses greater than average in number** (Goldfried et al., 1971; Kahn & Giffen, 1960; Miale & Harrower-Erickson, 1940; Ross & Ross, 1944; Schafer, 1948).
3. **Aggressive animal content with high form level** (Levi, 1951).
4. **Food content emphasized** (Phillips & Smith, 1953; Schafer, 1948; Wiener, 1956).
5. **Plant or botany content emphasized** (Kahn & Giffen, 1960).

Other Rorschach Indices
1. **Popular responses in greater than average quantity** (Beck, 1960; Berkowitz & Levine, 1953; Bradway & Heisler, 1953; Hertz, 1948; Mundy, 1972; Piotrowski, 1957; Rapaport et al., 1946).
2. **Popular responses in subnormal quantity** (Allen, 1954; Cox & Sarason, 1954; Fisher, 1950; Goldfried et al., 1971; Neuringer, 1962; Schwartz & Kates, 1957).
3. **Number of responses unusually small** (Alcock, 1963; Eichler, 1951; Fisher, 1950, 1951; Goldfried et al., 1971; Hertz, 1948, 1949; Holt, 1968; Kahn & Giffen, 1960; Miale & Harrower-Erickson,

1940; Neuringer, 1962; Olch, 1971; Phillips & Smith, 1953; Schachtel, 1966; Schafer, 1948; Sherman, 1955; Wagner, 1973).
4. **More than one rejection, or failure, of an ink blot** (Alcock, 1963; Allen, 1954; Beck, 1960; Bohm, 1958; Carnes & Bates, 1971; Fisher, 1950; Goldfried et al., 1971; Hertz, 1948, 1949; Holt, 1968; Klopfer et al., 1954, 1956; Miale & Harrower-Erickson, 1940; Munroe, 1945; Rorschach, 1921/1951; Shatin, 1952; Wagner, 1973).
5. **Edging observed** (Allen, 1954; Baker, 1956; Beck, 1945; Klopfer et al., 1954; Phillips & Smith, 1953).
6. **Rotating cards immediately on presentation** (Beck, 1945).
7. **Excessive card turning, especially when turned rapidly** (Beck, 1945).
8. **Blocking or shock to Card II** (Alcock, 1963; Ames et al., 1959, 1971; Beck & Molish, 1967; Goldfried et al., 1971; Hertz, 1948; Klopfer et al., 1954; Miale & Harrower-Erickson, 1940; Molish, 1967; Munroe, 1945; Phillips & Smith, 1953; Piotrowski, 1957; Schachtel, 1943, 1966).
9. **Spinning top to center** *S* **in Card II** (Lindner, 1950).
10. **Dislike for Card II, due to its association with blood** (Wallen, 1948).
11. **Shock to Card III** (Klopfer et al., 1954; Piotrowski, 1957; Piotrowski & Dudek, 1956).
12. **Shock to Card IV** (Ames et al., 1971; Bohm, 1960; Goldfried et al., 1971; Schachtel, 1966).
13. **Shock to Card VI** (Goldfried et al., 1971; Klopfer et al., 1954; Phillips & Smith, 1953; Piotrowski, 1957; Ross & Ross, 1944).
14. **Shock to Card VII** (Allen, 1954; Klopfer et al., 1954; Piotrowski, 1957; Ross & Ross, 1944).
15. **Marked blocking or shock to Card IX** (Ogdon, 1975; Ross & Ross, 1944).
16. **Shock to Card VIII** (Schachtel, 1966).
17. **No Animal Object Popular to Card VI** (Molish, 1951).

Projective Drawing Signs
Graphological and General Indices
1. **Excessive detailing** (Buck, 1948, 1964, 1966; Deabler, 1969; Hammer, 1954c, 1958, 1965, 1969a, 1969b; Jacks, 1969; Kahn & Giffen, 1960; Levy, 1958; Machover, 1949; McElhaney, 1969).
2. **Excessive erasing** (Kahn & Giffen, 1960; Machover, 1949; Urban, 1963).
3. **Very light pressure** (Hammer, 1954c, 1958; Handler & Reyher, 1966; Jolles, 1971; Machover, 1955; Precker, 1950; Urban, 1963).

4. **Very small drawings** (Brick, 1944; McHugh, 1966).
5. **Random scribbled shading** (Kahn & Giffen, 1960; Schildkrout et al., 1972).

Draw-A-Person/Human Figure Drawing Indices
1. **Head of drawing not given most attention** (Ogdon, 1975).
2. **Extreme bilateral symmetry** (Hammer, 1958; Machover, 1949; Modell & Potter, 1949; Urban, 1963).
3. **Marked asymmetry** (Koppitz, 1966c, 1968; Machover, 1949; McElhaney, 1969; Mundy, 1972; Rosenzweig & Kogan, 1949; Urban, 1963).
4. **Head drawn unusually large** (Hammer, 1954c; Machover, 1949; Schildkrout et al., 1972; Urban, 1963).
5. **Head drawn unusually small** (Buck, 1964, 1966; Gilbert, 1969; Machover, 1949; Jolles, 1971; Urban, 1963).
6. **Pupils omitted from eyes** (Hammer, 1954c, 1958, 1968; Kahn & Giffen, 1960; Levine & Sapolsky, 1969; Machover, 1949; Schildkrout et al., 1972; Urban, 1963).
7. **Legs pressed closely together** (Machover, 1949; Schildkrout et al., 1972; Urban, 1963).
8. **Small, especially tiny feet** (Brown, 1958; Buck, 1964, 1966, 1969; DiLeo, 1973; Jolles, 1971; Machover, 1949; Modell & Potter, 1949; Urban, 1963).

H-T-P House and Tree Drawing Indices
1. **House drawn very small** (Buck, 1948).
2. **Tree drawn as a dead tree** (Hammer, 1955, 1958).
3. **Long tree trunks with small crowns** (Koch, 1952).

Bender-Gestalt Signs
Unusual Reproduction Modes and Arrangements
1. **Closure difficulty** (Billingslea, 1948; Byrd, 1956; Clawson, 1959, 1962; Guertin, 1952; Hutt, 1953; Hutt & Briskin, 1960; Hutt & Gibby, 1970; Koppitz, 1958).
2. **Curvature modified significantly** (Billingslea, 1948; Guertin, 1952, 1954a, 1954b; Halpern, 1951; Hutt, 1953, 1977; Weiner, 1966).
3. **Fragmentation** (Gobetz, 1953; Hutt, 1953, 1968, 1977; Hutt & Briskin, 1960).
4. **Numbering and boxing of figures** (Billingslea, 1948; Gilbert, 1969; Gobetz, 1953; Lerner, 1972; Woltmann, 1950).
5. **Overlapping and crossing difficulty** (Byrd, 1956; Guertin, 1952; Hutt, 1953, 1977; Hutt & Briskin, 1960; Hutt & Gibby, 1970; Koppitz, 1958).

6. **Regression, including simplification, primitivation, and condensation** (Billingslea, 1948; Halpern, 1951; Hutt & Gibby, 1970).
7. **Reversals** (Hutt, 1953).
8. **Rotations** (Billingslea, 1948; Griffith & Taylor, 1960; Hutt & Briskin, 1960; Hutt & Gibby, 1970).
9. **Sketching** (Billingslea, 1948; Hutt, 1953).
10. **Excessive workover** (Billingslea, 1948; Gilbert, 1969).
11. **Spontaneous elaborations, embellishments and doodling** (Hutt & Briskin, 1960).
12. **Tremors and motor incoordination** (Tucker & Spielberg, 1958).
13. **Reduced size of reproductions, though Figure 4 may not be reduced** (Billingslea, 1948; Hutt, 1953, 1977).
14. **Confused or chaotic arrangement** (Gobetz, 1953).
15. **Sequential expansion of reproductions** (Hutt & Briskin, 1960).
16. **Rotation of stimulus card** (Hutt, 1977).
17. **Scattered, expansive arrangement** (Hutt & Briskin, 1960; Woltmann, 1950).
18. **Crowded, compressed, or cohesive arrangements** (Billingslea, 1948; Halpern, 1951; Hutt & Briskin, 1960; Woltmann, 1950).
19. **Rigidly methodical arrangements** (Hutt, 1953, 1977; Hutt & Briskin, 1960; Woltmann, 1950).
20. **Irregularity of figure size, line quality, or sequence** (Hutt, 1977).

Unusual Treatment of Specific Figures
1. **Overlapping of the two components of Figure A** (Billingslea, 1948).
2. **General difficulty with Figure 1** (Hutt & Briskin, 1960).
3. **Upward sloping on Figure 2** (Gobetz, 1953).
4. **Overlapping on Figure 4 due to bringing the parts too close together** (Billingslea, 1948).
5. **Enlargement of open square on Figure 4** (Billingslea, 1948).
6. **Counting dots repeatedly on Figure 5** (Gobetz, 1953; Hutt & Briskin, 1960; Lerner, 1972; Story, 1960; Weissman & Roth, 1965).
7. **Decreasing the amplitude of curves on Figure 6** (Billingslea, 1948; Gobetz, 1953).
8. **Excessive waves on Figure 6** (Gobetz, 1953; Guertin, 1952).
9. **Increased size of the angle on the left side of the hexagon in Figure 8** (Billingslea, 1948).
10. **Abnormal placement of Figure A** (Hutt, 1977).

ANXIETY

Anxiety is an emotional condition or affect which is fundamentally unpleasant. Spielberger (1972) more completely describes anxiety as "an unpleasant emotional state or condition which is characterized by subjective feelings of tension, apprehension, and worry, and by activation or arousal of the autonomic nervous system" (p. 482). Many forms of anxiety have been described. These include such diverse examples as id anxiety, ego anxiety, signal anxiety, castration anxiety, free-floating anxiety, ictal anxiety, primal anxiety, separation anxiety, and trait and state anxiety. These various uses of the term reflect the fact that there is not a single, universally accepted definition of anxiety. In current psychological literature three of these uses predominate: anxiety that is free-floating and is distinguished from fears and phobias, and trait and state anxiety.

Free-floating anxiety is an intense though vague, objectless fearful kind of feeling. Subjectively it is non-specific with regard to any internal or external sign or situation. The individual may be overwhelmed by the fearful apprehension though unable to explain or account for it. No cause can be singled out. Unless otherwise qualified, this is the meaning of anxiety used in this book. Fear, on the other hand, is specific and is related or attached to particular objects, signs, situations, or experiences which are in one's awareness. An individual will consciously avoid feared objects or situations whereas this is not possible in the case of anxiety. Phobias are pathognomonic, exaggerated, irrational fears. These, too, may be incapacitating or at least cause a significant decrement in the quality of adjusting of the individual when he or she is in the presence of the stimulus of the phobia.

Trait anxiety refers to a chronic chracteristic of an individual. It is durable apprehensiveness or high level of disquietude which persists more or less regardless of the situation. *State anxiety* refers to an acute, usually short-lived experience. It is situationally induced, and in state anxiety experiments the stimuli inducing the apprehension are largely under the control of the experimenter. Both state and trait anxiety are related to free-floating anxiety though neither is coincidental with it. As we have defined it, anxiety is episodic and acute, yet recurring and in a sense durable. In sum, anxiety should be considered as a panic type of "response to some as yet unrecognized factor, either in the environment or in the self" (Rycroft, 1973).

Behavioral Manifestations

Behavioral manifestations of anxiety are largely associated with sympathetic dominance of the autonomic nervous system. They include increased pulse, sweating, flushing, trembling, shortness of breath, insomnia, attacks of diarrhea, and in the extreme, a loss of continence as in enuresis and encopresis (cf. Coleman, 1972; Hinsie & Campbell, 1970). Inasmuch as anxiety and tension frequently are concomitant and their symptomatic expressions intermingled, reference should be made to the manifestations of tension (see next section in this chapter).

Test Indices

Wechsler Signs

1. **Unusually low Digit Span scores** (Allison, 1978; Allison et al., 1968; Blatt, 1965; Gilbert, 1969; Glasser & Zimmerman, 1967; Gurvitz, 1951; Harrower, 1956; Holt, 1968; Kaufman, 1979; Lewinski, 1945; Mayman et al., 1951; Moldawsky & Moldawsky, 1952; Patterson, 1953; Pope & Scott, 1967; Rapaport et al., 1945; Schafer, 1948; Siegman, 1956; Walker & Spence, 1964; Wechsler, 1958; Zimmerman & Woo-Sam, 1973).

2. **Unusually low Information scores** (Allison et al., 1968; Gilbert, 1969; Glasser & Zimmerman, 1967; Holt, 1968; Lanfeld & Saunders, 1961; Rapaport et al., 1945; Schafer, 1948).

3. **Unusually low Arithmetic scores** (Gilbert, 1969; Glasser & Zimmerman, 1967; Harrower, 1956; Kaufman, 1979; Schafer, 1948; Siegman, 1956; Wechsler, 1958; Zimmerman & Woo-Sam, 1973).

4. **Digit Span significantly below Arithmetic** (Ogdon, 1975).

5. **Arithmetic and Digit Span scores both unusually low** (Allison et al., 1968; Kaufman, 1979).

6. **Unusually low Picture Completion score** (Glasser & Zimmerman, 1967; Gurvitz, 1951; Lanfeld & Saunders, 1961; Zimmerman & Woo-Sam, 1973).

7. **Unusually low Object Assembly score** (Allison et al., 1968; Blatt, Allison, & Baker, 1965; Gilbert, 1969; Glasser & Zimmerman, 1967; Gurvitz, 1951; Holt, 1968; Lanfeld & Saunders, 1961; Mayman et al., 1951; Rapaport et al., 1945; Schafer, 1948; Siegman, 1956; Zimmerman & Woo-Sam, 1973).

8. **Unusually low Block Design score** (Allison, 1978; Allison et al., 1968; Blatt, 1965; Glasser & Zimmerman, 1967; Mayman et al., 1951; Rashkis & Welsh, 1946; Siegman, 1956; Schafer, 1948; Zimmerman & Woo-Sam, 1973).

9. **Unusually low Digit Symbol or Coding score** (Allison, 1978; Gilbert, 1969; Kaufman, 1979; Ladd, 1964; Mandler & Sarason, 1951; Patterson, 1953; Siegman, 1956; Solkoff, 1964; Solkoff & Chrisien, 1963; Wechsler, 1958).

10. **Verbal IQ significantly above Performance IQ** (Gurvitz, 1951; Maley, 1970; Mayman et al., 1951; Pope & Scott, 1967; Schafer, 1948; Wechsler, 1958; Zimmerman & Woo-Sam, 1973).

Rorschach Signs
Indices Utilizing Determinants

1. **Greater than normal number of shading responses** (Acker, 1963; Allen, 1954; Allison et al., 1968; Auerbach & Spielberger, 1972; Beck, 1960; Bochner & Halpern, 1945; Eichler, 1951; Exner, 1974; Halpern, 1953; Hertz, 1948, 1949, 1960; Kahn & Giffen, 1960; Klopfer et al., 1954; Rickers-Ovsiankina, 1960; Rosenzweig & Kogan, 1949; Sarason, 1954; Schachtel, 1943, 1966; Schwartz & Kates, 1957; Wagner, 1971; Wagner & Slemboski, 1969; Waller, 1960a, 1960b).

2. **Greater than normal number of diffuse, *KF* and *K* type responses** (Acker, 1963; Alcock, 1963; Allen, 1954, 1958; Arnaud, 1959; Beck, 1951; Beck & Molish, 1967; Bochner & Halpern, 1945; Gurvitz, 1951; Hafner & Rosen, 1964; Halpern, 1953; Hertz, 1948; Klopfer & Davidson, 1962; Lebo, Toal, & Brick, 1960; Levitt, 1957; Levitt & Grosz, 1960; Mons, 1950; Sarason, 1954; Schafer, 1948; Waller, 1960a).

3. **Greater than normal number of Vista responses** (Allen, 1954; Beck, 1945; Bochner & Halpern, 1945; Brar, 1970; Ferguson, 1952; Hertz, 1948; Klopfer & Davidson, 1962; Molish, 1967; Phillips & Smith, 1953; Waller, 1960a).

4. **Greater than normal number of surface shading, texture, *Fc* type responses** (Acker, 1963; Ames et al., 1952, 1959; Arnaud, 1959; Beck, 1951, 1960; Bochner & Halpern, 1945; Cox & Sarason, 1954; Eichler, 1951; Goodstein & Goldberger, 1955; Halpern, 1953; Hertz, 1948, 1949; Klopfer & Kelley, 1942; Levitt, 1957; Molish, 1967; Neuringer, 1962; Piotrowski, 1957; Rapaport et al., 1946; Sarason, 1954; Wagner, 1971; Waller, 1960a, 1960b; Zelen, 1970).

5. **Subnormal number of surface shading, texture, *Fc* type of responses** (Cox & Sarason, 1954; Piotrowski, 1957; Rapaport et al., 1946; Sarason, 1954; Schwartz & Kates, 1957).

6. **Shading used to depict three dimensions projected onto a two-dimensional plane; X-ray, *Fk*, *kF* and *k* type of responses in greater than normal numbers** (Allen, 1954; Arnaud, 1959; Beck, 1951; Gurvitz, 1951; Halpern, 1953; Hertz, 1948; Klopfer et al., 1954; Klopfer & Davidson, 1962; Munroe, 1950).

7. **$FK + Fc$ greater than 75% of *F*** (Allison et al., 1968; Eichler, 1951; Klopfer & Davidson, 1962).

8. **Poor quality Vista responses present** (Hertz, 1948).

9. **$F\%$ greater than 50** (Kates, 1950; Kates & Schwartz, 1958; Klopfer et al., 1954; Lord, 1950; Neuringer, 1962; Perdue, 1964; Rapaport et al., 1946; Riessman & Miller, 1958; Schwartz & Kates, 1957; Singer, 1960).

10. **Subnormal quality of *F* responses** (Arnaud, 1959; Baker & Harris, 1949; Cox & Sarason, 1954; Eichler, 1951; Holt, 1968; Korchin, 1960; Levitt & Grosz, 1960; Phillips & Smith, 1953; Piotrowski, 1957; Rapaport et al., 1946; Sarason, 1954; Schafer, 1948).

11. **Subnormal number of *M* responses** (Affleck & Mednick, 1959; Auerbach & Spielberger, 1972; Beck, 1960; Bohm, 1958; Fisher, 1951; Hertz, 1948; Kates & Schwartz, 1958; Neuringer, 1962; Phillips & Smith, 1953; Rapaport et al., 1946; Riessman & Miller, 1958; Schafer, 1948; Schwartz & Kates, 1957).

12. **Poor quality *M* responses** (Beck, 1978; Levitt & Grosz, 1960).

13. ***M* responses with (*H*) content** (Phillips & Smith, 1953).

14. ***M* responses with *Hd* content** (Phillips & Smith, 1953).

15. ***FM* responses in greater than normal number** (Adams et al., 1963; Cox & Sarason, 1954; Levitt & Grosz, 1960).

16. **Inanimate movement responses in greater than normal number** (Allen, 1954, 1958; Ames et al., 1952, 1959, 1971; Arnaud, 1959; Bochner & Halpern, 1945; Cox & Sarason, 1954; Hafner & Rosen, 1964; Hertz, 1960; Hertz & Paolino, 1960; Kahn & Giffen, 1960; Kates & Schwartz, 1958; Klopfer & Davidson, 1962; Levitt & Truumaa, 1972; Meyer, 1961; Neel, 1960; Neuringer, 1962; Phillips & Smith, 1953; Piotrowski, 1937a, 1957; Schwartz & Kates, 1957; Wagner, 1971; Zelen, 1970).

17. **Inanimate movement responses with frightening or precariously balanced content** (Arnaud, 1959).

18. ***FC* determinants subnormal in number** (Fisher, 1950; Goldfried et al., 1971; Hertz, 1948; Kahn & Giffen, 1960; Kates, 1950; Miale & Harrower-Erickson, 1940; Munroe, 1945; Piotrowski, 1957; Rapaport et al., 1946).

19. ***CF* determinants in greater than normal number** (Sarason, 1954).

20. ***CF* + *C* approximately zero in number** (Klopfer & Davidson, 1962; Neuringer, 1962; Piotrowski,

1957; Piotrowski & Dudek, 1956; Schafer, 1954; Shapiro, 1960).

21. *FC + CF + C* **approximately zero in number** (Bohm, 1958; Kates, 1950; Riessman & Miller, 1958).

22. **Achromatic determinants used in greater than normal number** (Ames et al., 1952; Arnaud, 1959; Beck, 1951, 1960; Bohm, 1960; Hertz, 1948; Piotrowski, 1957; Rapaport et al., 1946; Rosenzweig & Kogan, 1949; Rorschach, 1921/1951; Wagner, 1971).

23. **Pure *C* or crude *C* responses present** (Fisher, 1950; Goldfried et al., 1971; Phillips & Smith, 1953).

24. **Presence of *c* responses** (Allen, 1954; Halpern, 1953; Levitt, 1957; Levitt & Grosz, 1960; Neuringer, 1962; Piotrowski, 1957; Schafer, 1948, 1954; Wagner, 1971).

25. **Sum *C* greater than 3** (Haworth, 1962; Hertz, 1948; Murstein, 1960; Rapaport et al., 1946).

Indices Utilizing Locations

1. *D* **locations used in greater than normal number** (Beck, 1945; Klopfer & Davidson, 1962).

2. *W* **locations used in greater than normal number** (Goodstein & Goldberger, 1955; Kates & Schwartz, 1958; Lucas, 1961; Phillips & Smith, 1953; Schafer, 1954).

3. *W* **locations subnormal in number** (Bohm, 1958; Cox & Sarason, 1954; Doris et al., 1963; Eichler, 1951; Exner, 1974; Levitt & Grosz, 1960; Neuringer, 1962; Phillips & Smith, 1953; Rapaport et al., 1946; Riessman & Miller, 1958; Sarason, 1954; Schachtel, 1966; Schafer, 1954; Schwartz & Kates, 1957).

4. **Cut off *W* locations used in greater than normal number** (Phillips & Smith, 1953).

5. *Dd* **locations emphasized** (Ames et al., 1952, 1974; Davidson, 1950; Doris et al., 1963; Hammes & Osborne, 1962; Holt, 1968; Klopfer et al., 1954; Piotrowski, 1957; Sarason, 1954; Schachtel, 1966).

6. **Small common detail, *d*-type locations used in greater than normal number** (Gurvitz, 1951; Halpern, 1953; Klopfer & Davidson, 1962; Levitt & Truumaa, 1972; Piotrowski, 1957; Schafer, 1954).

7. *Dd + S* **locations used in greater than normal number** (Ames et al., 1952, 1974; Davidson, 1950; Hammes & Osborne, 1962; Klopfer et al., 1954).

8. *di* **responses emphasized** (Alcock, 1963; Bochner & Halpern, 1945; Klopfer & Davidson, 1962).

9. *de* **locations emphasized** (Bochner & Halpern, 1945; Klopfer & Davidson, 1962; Rapaport et al., 1946).

10. *do* **locations used** (Allen, 1954; Allison et al., 1968; Ames et al., 1952, 1974; Auerbach & Spielberger, 1972; Beck, 1945; Bochner & Halpern, 1945; Bohm, 1958; Eichler, 1951; Holt, 1968; Piotrowski, 1957; Rapaport et al., 1946; Rorschach, 1921/1951; Sarason, 1954).

Indices Utilizing Content Categories

1. *Hd* **used in greater than normal number** (Ames et al., 1952, 1959; Beck, 1978; Phillips & Smith, 1953; Piotrowski, 1957; Rapaport et al., 1946).

2. **(*H*) used in greater than normal number** (DeVos, 1952; Phillips & Smith, 1953).

3. **Sophisticated anatomy and X-ray content present in significant number** (Allen, 1954; Brar, 1970; Lindner, 1946; Phillips & Smith, 1953).

4. **Weird or bizarre concepts such as mummies, giants, cadavers, deformed or dying animals, etc., present in significant number** (Ames, 1959; Arnaud, 1959; Beck, 1960; DeVos, 1952; Elizur, 1949; Goldfried, 1966a; Goldfried et al., 1971; Haworth, 1962; Kagan, 1960; Neuringer, 1962).

5. **Blood content used in greater than normal number** (Beck, 1978; Brar, 1970; DeVos, 1952; Elizur, 1949; Goldfried, 1966a; Haworth, 1962; Lindner, 1946; Phillips & Smith, 1953).

6. **Alphabet, numbers, punctuation, and geometric figure content present in significant number** (Arnaud, 1959; Halpern, 1953).

7. **Crude anatomy content present** (Lindner, 1946; Pope & Scott, 1967).

8. **Anatomy content used in greater than normal number** (Allen, 1954; Allison et al., 1968; Elizur, 1949; Goldfried, 1966a; Neuringer, 1962; Rav, 1951; Sandler & Acker, 1951; Wagner, 1961).

9. **Animal content used in greater than normal number** (Beck, 1945; Phillips & Smith, 1953; Piotrowski, 1957).

10. *Hdx* **and *Adx* content present in significant numbers** (Allen, 1954; Beck, 1944, 1945, 1978; Phillips & Smith, 1953).

11. *Ad* **content used in greater than normal number** (Allen, 1954; Bochner & Halpern, 1945; Piotrowski, 1957; Rorschach, 1921/1951).

12. **Cloud content used in greater than normal number** (Allen, 1954; Brar, 1970; DeVos, 1952; Elizur, 1949; Goldfried, 1966a).

13. **Fire content used in greater than normal number** (Brar, 1970; Elizur, 1949; Goldfried, 1966a; Palmer, 1970; Phillips & Smith, 1953; Rychlak & Guinouard, 1961).

14. **Smoke content present in significant number** (Brar, 1970; DeVos, 1952; Elizur, 1949; Goldfried, 1966a; Phillips & Smith, 1953; Schafer, 1954).

15. **Map content used in greater than normal number** (Allen, 1954; Brar, 1970; DeVos, 1952).

16. **H + A less than twice Hd + Ad** (Allen, 1954; Ames et al., 1959, 1971; Beck, 1945; Bochner & Halpern, 1945; Bohm, 1958; Klopfer & Davidson, 1962; Phillips & Smith, 1953; Piotrowski, 1957; Potkay, 1971; Rorschach, 1921/1951).

17. **Subnormal number of content categories used** (Allen, 1958; Allison et al., 1968; Beck, 1945; Hertz, 1948, 1949; Munroe, 1945; Piotrowski, 1969; Schachtel, 1966).

18. **AHybrid, a combination of A, H, and/or Plant content present** (DeVos, 1952).

19. **Any dangerous or frightening place or action described** (DeVos, 1952; Elizur, 1949; Goldfried, 1966a).

Other Rorschach Indices

1. **Unusually small number of responses** (Alcock, 1963; Hertz, 1948, 1949; Eichler, 1951; Fisher, 1950, 1951; Goldfried et al., 1971; Holt, 1968; Kahn & Giffen, 1960; Miale & Harrower-Erickson, 1940; Neuringer, 1962; Olch, 1971; Phillips & Smith, 1953; Schachtel, 1966; Schafer, 1948; Sherman, 1955; Wagner, 1973).

2. **Popular responses subnormal in number** (Allen, 1954; Cox & Sarason, 1954; Fisher, 1950; Goldfried et al., 1971; Neuringer, 1962; Schwartz & Kates, 1957).

3. **Popular responses present in greater than normal number** (Neuringer, 1962).

4. **Perseverations and repetitions present** (Arnaud, 1959; Cox & Sarason, 1954; Evans & Marmorston, 1963, 1964; Sarason, 1954).

5. **More than one rejection or failure** (Arnaud, 1959; Beck, 1960; DeVos, 1952; Kahn & Giffen, 1960; Kaswan, Wasman, & Freedman, 1960; Kates, 1950; Klopfer et al., 1954; Neuringer, 1962; Schwartz & Kates, 1957).

6. **Refusing to take Rorschach cards in hand** (Phillips & Smith, 1953).

7. **Excessive qualifications of responses** (Beck, 1945).

8. **Unpleasant dysphoric tone or emotions expressed in responses** (Arnaud, 1959; DeVos, 1952; Elizur, 1949; Goldfried et al., 1971).

9. **Number of responses is greater than normal** (Alcock, 1963; Siegal et al., 1962).

10. **Reaction and response times unusually long** (Allen, 1954; Auerbach & Spielberger, 1972; Cox & Sarason, 1954; Goodstein & Goldberger, 1955; Harris, 1960; Holt, 1968; Kahn & Giffen, 1960; Lebo et al., 1960; Levitt & Grosz, 1960; Meyer & Caruth, 1970; Neuringer, 1962; Schwartz & Kates, 1957).

11. **Reaction times unusually short** (Cox & Sarason, 1954).

12. **Spinning top to center S on Card II** (Lindner, 1950).

13. **Shock to Card IV** (Allen, 1954; Beck, 1960; Beck & Molish, 1967; Beck et al., 1961; Bohm, 1958, 1960, 1977; Hertz, 1949; Klopfer et al., 1954; Molish, 1967; Phillips & Smith, 1953).

14. **Shock to Card VI** (Goldfried et al., 1971; Klopfer et al., 1954; Molish, 1967; Phillips & Smith, 1953; Piotrowski, 1957).

15. **Blocking to Plate II** (Beck, 1978; Beck & Molish, 1967; Beck et al., 1961).

Projective Drawing Signs
Graphological and General Indices

1. **Excessive shading and shaded strokes** (Allen, 1958; Buck, 1948, 1964, 1966; Deabler, 1969; DiLeo, 1970, 1973; Exner, 1962; Hammer, 1954c, 1958, 1969a, 1978; Handler & Reyher, 1966; Jacks, 1969; Jolles, 1969, 1971; Landisberg, 1958; Levy, 1950, 1958; Machover, 1949, 1951, 1958; Reynolds, 1978; Schildkrout et al., 1972; Urban, 1963; Wolk, 1969; Wysocki & Whitney, 1965).

2. **Very short, circular, shaky or sketchy strokes** (Buck, 1964; DeCato & Wicks, 1976; Gurvitz, 1951; Hammer, 1958; Jolles, 1971; Levy, 1950, 1958; Urban, 1963).

3. **Vague lines, vacillating in direction or with interrupted strokes** (Hammer, 1954c; Jacks, 1969; Levy, 1950, 1958; Wolff, 1946).

4. **Excessive detailing** (Buck, 1948, 1964, 1966; Deabler, 1969; Goldstein & Faterson, 1969; Hammer, 1954c, 1958, 1965, 1969a, 1969b; Jacks, 1969; Kahn & Giffen, 1960; Levy, 1958; Machover, 1949; McElhaney, 1969).

5. **Jagged lines and edges** (Hammer, 1965; Krout, 1950; Machover, 1951; Urban, 1963; Waehner, 1946).

6. **Very light pressure** (DeCato & Wicks, 1976; Hammer, 1954c, 1958; Handler & Reyher, 1966; Hutt, 1977; Jolles, 1971; Machover, 1955; Precker, 1950; Saarni & Azara, 1977; Urban, 1963).

7. **Very heavy pressure** (Deabler, 1969; DeCato & Wicks, 1976; Hammer, 1969a; Handler & Reyher, 1964, 1965, 1966; Reynolds, 1978).

26

8. **Excessive erasing** (Allen, 1958; Jacks, 1969; Machover, 1949).

9. **Very small drawings** (DeCato & Wicks, 1976; Hammer, 1968, 1978; Hoyt & Baron, 1959; Kadis, 1950; Rosenzweig & Kogan, 1949; Saarni & Azara, 1977; Waehner, 1946).

10. **Upper left-hand corner placement** (Barnouw, 1969; Buck, 1948; Hoyt & Baron, 1959; Johnson, 1971; Jolles, 1971; Urban, 1963).

11. **Edge or bottom placement** (Hutt, 1977; Jolles, 1952a).

12. **Moderate distortions in drawing** (Handler & Reyher, 1965, 1966).

13. **Omission of important or essential details** (Mogar, 1962; Reynolds, 1978).

14. **Very heavy groundlines** (Jolles, 1971).

15. **Shadows spontaneously drawn in projective drawings** (Hammer, 1954c; Jolles, 1971).

Draw-A-Person/Human Figure Drawing Indices

1. **Unusually large head** (Mogar, 1962; Wysocki & Whitney, 1965).

2. **Hair heavily shaded** (Jolles, 1971; Mogar, 1962; Urban, 1963).

3. **Eyes that are abnormally large or strongly reinforced, especially if shaded** (Machover, 1958), **or are strabismic (cross-eyed or walleyed)** (Saarni & Azara, 1977).

4. **Arms unequal in length** (Gurvitz, 1951; Saarni & Azara, 1977).

5. **Hands drawn with significant shading** (Buck, 1964; Jolles, 1971; Koppitz, 1968; Levy, 1950, 1958; Machover, 1949; Urban, 1963).

6. **Shading of same sex human figure drawing** (Goldstein & Faterson, 1969).

7. **Drawing opposite sex first** (Klopfer & Taulbee, 1976).

8. **Omission of any of the following: arms, hands, fingers, eyes, mouth, neck, legs, feet, or shoes** (Saarni & Azara, 1977).

9. **Arms that are very large, very short, or clinging to the side of the body** (Saarni & Azara, 1977).

10. **Person drawing that is very large, less than 3″ high, or slanting more than 15 degrees** (Saarni & Azara, 1977).

11. **Transparencies present** (Handler & Reyher, 1965; Saarni & Azara, 1977).

12. **Very large fingers or hands drawn** (Saarni & Azara, 1977).

House and Tree Drawing Indices

1. **Shadows are cast by the House** (Hammer, 1954c; Jacks, 1969).

2. **Clouds spontaneously added to House drawing** (Hammer, 1954c; Jacks, 1969).

3. **Chimney smoking in great profusion** (Buck, 1948, 1964, 1966; Hammer, 1958; Jolles, 1971).

4. **Emphasis on baseline to the wall** (Jolles, 1971).

5. **Very faint branches on Tree drawing** (Buck, 1948).

6. **Bark that is inconsistently drawn or heavily reinforced** (Buck, 1966; Jolles, 1971).

7. **Tree roots significantly shaded** (Michal-Smith & Morgenstern, 1969).

8. **Shadows are cast by the Tree** (Jolles, 1971).

9. **Tree drawing with a very faint trunk** (Buck, 1964, 1966; Jolles, 1971).

Bender-Gestalt Signs

Unusual Reproduction Modes and Arrangements

1. **Angulation changes** (Halpern, 1951).

2. **Closure difficulty** (Clawson, 1962; Halpern, 1951; Hutt & Gibby, 1970).

3. **Fragmentation** (Gobetz, 1953; Hutt, 1953, 1968; Hutt & Briskin, 1960).

4. **Reduced size of reproductions** (Gavales & Millon, 1960; Hutt, 1953, 1968, 1978; Hutt & Briskin, 1960).

5. **Sketching** (Clawson, 1962; Halpern, 1951; Hutt, 1953; Hutt & Briskin, 1960; Koppitz, 1958).

6. **Spontaneous elaborations, embellishments, and doodling** (Hutt, 1977; Hutt & Briskin, 1960).

7. **Tremors and motor incoordination** (Curnutt, 1953; Hutt, 1953, 1977; Pascal & Suttell, 1951; Zolik, 1958).

8. **Excessive workover** (Billingslea, 1948; Gilbert, 1969).

9. **Confused, compressed, and chaotic arrangements** (Hutt, 1953, 1968, 1978; Hutt & Briskin, 1960; Koppitz, 1958).

10. **Rigidly methodical arrangements** (Halpern, 1951).

Unusual Treatment of Specific Figures

1. **Separation of open square from curved line on Figure A** (Halpern, 1951; Lerner, 1972), **or Figure A is very small** (Hutt, 1977).

2. **General difficulty with Figure 1** (Hutt, 1977; Hutt & Briskin, 1960).

3. **Dots or lines substituted for circles on Figure 2** (Hutt, 1968, 1977; Hutt & Briskin, 1960).

4. **Sketching, reinforcing lines, heavy lines, and particularly inaccurately relating the two parts on Figure 4** (Suczek & Klopfer, 1952).

5. **Sketching, redrawing, and erasures on Figure 8** (Suczek & Klopfer, 1952).

6. **Increased angular relationship on Figure 6** (De-Cato & Wicks, 1976).

Contraindications

1. **W+ responses on the Rorschach** (Bochner & Halpern, 1945; Holt, 1968).
2. **Absence of shading responses on the Rorschach** (Klopfer et al., 1954; Wagner, 1971).
3. **Unusually high Digit Span and Block Design scores** (Allison, 1978).

TENSION

The expressions "nervous tension," "emotional tension," and "social tension" are used in various contexts by professionals and nonprofessionals alike (cf. English & English, 1958; Webster's New World Dictionary, 1976). In fact, where literal tension exists in the use of these terms, it is muscular tension. Nervous tension, at bottom, is a feeling of distress. It does not refer to taut nerves because nerves are not strained or tense in the narrow sense but rather simply transmitting neural impulses. Certainly nerves activate the musculature, and ideas stored in the central nervous system may cause the experience of being "uptight" or "under pressure"—colloquialisms expressing a feeling of tension. Except for the epiphenomenon of tightening some muscles (as in clenching teeth with jaw muscles), the psychological concept of tension is largely metaphorical. Conflict and frustration are the basic causes, and they may be clearly conscious, unconscious, or somewhere in between.

A marked experience of tension is one of the general symptoms of the neuroses and the psychosomatic or psychophysiologic disorders. Many psychotics, on the other hand, have freed themselves from this distressful and disquieting symptom by virtue of their loss of contact with reality.

Behavioral Manifestations

Behavioral manifestations of tension include an increase in muscular tautness, particularly in the jaw and neck. There is an impaired ability to relax and one's appendages may actually be held rather tightly as opposed to a more normal lithe or limber state. The tendency toward muscular rigidity is a motoric manifestation of the neurotic's rather generalized loss of flexibility in adjusting. Other manifestations of tension are less obvious or relatively covert and tend to overlap those associated with anxiety, even as tension and anxiety often occur together. Some hold that tension is, at least in part, an expression of anxiety.

Test Indices

Wechsler Signs
1. **VIQ significantly above PIQ** (Gurvitz, 1951; Maley, 1970; Mayman et al., 1951; Pope & Scott, 1967; Schafer, 1948; Wechsler, 1958).
2. **Digit Span score unusually low** (Allison et al., 1968; Blatt, 1965; Glasser & Zimmerman, 1967; Gurvitz, 1951; Harrower, 1956; Holt, 1968; Lewinski, 1945; Mayman et al., 1951; Moldawsky & Moldawsky, 1952; Patterson, 1953; Pope & Scott, 1967; Rapaport et al., 1945; Schafer, 1948; Walker & Spence, 1964; Wechsler, 1958).
3. **Object Assembly score unusually low** (Allison et al., 1968; Blatt et al., 1965; Glasser & Zimmerman, 1967; Gurvitz, 1951; Holt, 1968; Lanfeld et al., 1961; Mayman et al., 1951; Rapaport et al., 1945; Schafer, 1948; Siegman, 1956).
4. **Digit Symbol score unusually low** (Mandler & Sarason, 1951; Patterson, 1953; Siegman, 1956; Solkoff, 1964; Solkoff & Chrisien, 1963).
5. **Block Design score unusually low** (Hardison & Purcell, 1959; Mayman et al., 1951; Rapaport et al., 1945).

Rorschach Signs
1. **Subnormal number of M responses** (Affleck & Mednick, 1959; Auerbach & Spielberger, 1972; Beck, 1960; Bohm, 1958; Fisher, 1951; Hertz, 1948; Kates & Schwartz, 1958; Neuringer, 1962; Phillips & Smith, 1953; Rapaport et al., 1946; Riessman & Miller, 1958; Schafer, 1948; Schwartz & Kates, 1957).
2. **M determinants with abstract content** (Miale, 1947; Phillips & Smith, 1953).
3. **Greater than normal number of inanimate movement responses** (Exner, 1974; Hertz, 1960; Klopfer & Davidson, 1962; Mayman, 1977; Neel, 1960; Phillips & Smith, 1953; Reisman, 1961; Spivack et al., 1959; Wagner, 1971).
4. **M greater than FM where FM is 1 or 0** (Klopfer et al., 1954).
5. **FM + m equal to or greater than 2M** (Klopfer & Davidson, 1962).
6. **Achromatic responses present in greater than normal number** (Ames et al., 1952, 1974; Arnaud, 1959; Beck, 1951, 1960; Bohm, 1960; Exner, 1974; Hertz, 1948; Piotrowski, 1957; Rapaport et al., 1946; Rorschach, 1921/1951; Rosenzweig & Kogan, 1949; Wagner, 1971).
7. **Cut off W responses present in significant number** (Phillips & Smith, 1953).

8. **Fire content emphasized** (Brar, 1970; Elizur, 1949; Palmer, 1970; Phillips & Smith, 1953; Rychlak & Guinouard, 1961).

Projective Drawing Signs

1. **Very heavy pressure used** (Buck, 1964; Hammer, 1958, 1968; Jolles, 1971; Kadis, 1950; Machover, 1955; Urban, 1963).
2. **Drawings done with extreme bilateral symmetry** (Hammer, 1958; Machover, 1949; Modell & Potter, 1949; Urban, 1963).
3. **Broken or reinforced waistline on figure drawing** (Machover, 1949; Modell & Potter, 1949).
4. **Stiff posture in drawn person** (Gilbert, 1969; Jacks, 1969; Schildkrout et al., 1972).
5. **Legs of figure drawing pressed closely together** (Buck, 1964; Jolles, 1969, 1971; Schildkrout et al., 1972; Urban, 1963).
6. **A very large, page-filling H-T-P House drawing** (Buck, 1948).
7. **H-T-P House drawn with chimney smoking in great profusion** (Buck, 1948, 1964, 1966; Hammer, 1958; Jolles, 1971).
8. **Peripheral wall lines to House drawing are faint and inadequate** (Hammer, 1958; Jolles, 1971).
9. **H-T-P Tree crown drawn with swirling heavy lines** (Landisberg, 1969).

Bender-Gestalt Signs

1. **Sketchy line quality** (Clawson, 1962; Halpern, 1951; Hutt, 1953; Hutt & Briskin, 1960; Koppitz, 1958).
2. **Tremors and motor incoordination manifested** (Curnutt, 1953; Hutt, 1953; Pascal & Suttell, 1951).
3. **Figure A drawn with irregular line quality** (Hutt, 1968).
4. **Heavy pressure used** (DeCato & Wicks, 1976).
5. **Dots enlarged** (DeCato & Wicks, 1976).
6. **Reproductions are made hastily** (Hutt, 1977).

TWO MODES OF NEUROTIC ADJUSTING

In 1967, Pope and Scott, in their excellent text *Psychological Diagnosis in Clinical Practice,* discussed how their clinical experience supports the position drawn from psychoanalytic theory that the neuroses exist along a dimension defined by hysterical repressiveness at one end of the continuum and obsessive intellectualization at the other. Other classical forms of neurosis, such as neurasthenia, are not even listed in their index. A perusal of Ogdon (1975) yields a paucity of test signs associated with those classical neuroses, although indices of anxiety and phobic tendencies have been catalogued there. These observations have led us to consider most neurotic conditions that are not anxiety or depressive neuroses as lying either in the repressive-hysterical or the intellectualizing obsessive-compulsive mode of adjusting. The dearth of test signs associated with other neuroses prevented extended consideration of them in separate sections of this volume.

An expression of these two neurotic modes was noted earlier by Levine and Spivack (1964) during the development of their Rorschach index of repressive style (RIRS). Their scale was devised so that "high RIRS scorers should be identified with the obsessive-intellectualizing end of the personality scale, and low scorers with the repressive-hysteric end" (p. 82). The psychological literature surveyed here suggests that this dimension of neurosis, clearly expressed in neurotics' speech, is also manifested in responses to other projective techniques as well as on the Wechsler scales (cf. Holt, 1968; Mayman & Cole, 1978).

Repression has been defined as "the process . . . by which an unacceptable impulse or idea is rendered unconscious" (Rycroft, 1973), or as "the exclusion of specific . . . activities or contents from conscious awareness by a process of which the individual is not directly aware" (English & English, 1958). *Hysteria* refers to a behavioral disorder characterized by mnemonic disturbances, a tendency toward dissociation, and sundry sensory, motor, and other somatic complaints for which there is no adequate physical basis. Analytic theory holds that the repressive process is the immediate psychodynamic cause of these symptoms, although symptom choice is complex and is influenced by numerous factors.

Basically, repressive-hysterical individuals may be characterized as spontaneous and impulsive. The impulsivity may be expressed in inaccuracy of responding as well as intellectual laziness (cf. Pope & Scott, 1967). They may be childish and dramatic in their affective lability. These proclivities ordinarily are readily observable in their psychological test responses as articulated below.

Intellectualization is a defense used to avoid affect and any unpleasant feeling which may accompany emotional arousal. It represents the use of logic, often implying a denial of ego-alien feeling associated with an idea or response tendency. *Obsessive-compulsive* patients report intruding ideas which are repetitive, distracting, and usually appear to be meaningless, even absurd or bizarre. These neurotics' behavior takes the form of compulsive, repetitive, stereotyped, ritualistic acts (cf. Rycroft, 1973). This behavior may have symbolic meaning and often is motivated to reduce anxiety associated with unconscious aspects of obsessive ideas. The defense of isolation is frequently brought to bear. In these instances the individual dissociates the affective component of ego-alien ideas or response tendencies and then rationalizes the idea or response tendency. Emotional bases or counterparts are divorced from the idea or propensity which continues in consciousness with the conscious residue explained on rational, intellectual, logical grounds. Isolation may be viewed as the obsessive's counterpart to the hysteric's straightforward repression. In isolation the dissociation occurs between an affective charge and the associated idea or memory. In fugue states and cases of multiple personality hysteria, dissociation occurs on a grand scale. In obsessives, the cognitive idea, wish, or mnemonic activity becomes divorced, due to repressive forces, from a strong, ego-alien affective load. The affect is lost from consciousness while the cognitive component remains in awareness (cf. English & English, 1958; Laughlin, 1979; Rycroft, 1973; Symonds, 1946).

REPRESSIVE-HYSTERICAL CONDITIONS

Behavioral Manifestations

Behavioral manifestations of hysterical conditions, in addition to the general behavioral manifestations of neuroses, include:

1. Fugue reactions in which the individual forgets (represses) his or her present identity and life situation, usually leaves his or her habitat for a new locale, and establishes a new identity and often a new life style (dissociative behavior).
2. Multiple personality actions in which the individual usually does not leave the locale but rather alternatingly acts with two or more relatively independent pseudo-identities and life styles (also dissociative behavior).
3. Amnesia for a protracted period of time which nevertheless is usually of shorter duration and without the other manifestations of a fugue. (Amnestic episodes are a type of temporary dissociative act.)
4. Behaving without the use of one or more sense modalities as in conversion blindness or deafness.
5. Acting without the use or with distorted use of certain muscles as in astasia abasia and other conversion paralyses.

More complete clinical descriptions of these individuals may be found in standard psychological texts (e.g., Allison, 1978; Coleman, 1972; Martin, 1977; Ullmann & Krasner, 1975).

Test Indices

Wechsler Signs

1. **Performance IQ significantly above the Verbal IQ** (Allison et al., 1968; Gilbert, 1969; Holt, 1968; Pope & Scott, 1967; Rabin & McKinney, 1972; Schafer, 1948; Zimmerman & Woo-Sam, 1973).
2. **Unusually low Information scores** (Allison et al., 1968; Blatt & Allison, 1968; Gilbert, 1969; Glasser & Zimmerman, 1967; Holt, 1968; Lanfeld & Saunders, 1961; Mayman et al., 1951; Pope & Scott, 1967; Rapaport et al., 1945; Schafer, 1948; Zimmerman & Woo-Sam, 1973).
3. **Information significantly below the Comprehension score** (Allison, 1978; Allison et al., 1968; Holt, 1968).
4. **Unusually low Arithmetic scores** (Allison et al., 1968; Blatt & Allison, 1968).
5. **Unusually low Arithmetic and Digit Span scores** (Allison et al., 1968).
6. **Unusually low Digit Symbol scores** (Gilbert, 1969; Ladd, 1964; Wechsler, 1958).
7. **Unusually low Block Design scores** (Glasser & Zimmerman, 1967).

Rorschach Signs

Determinant Indices

1. **Subnormal number of** *M* (Affleck & Mednick, 1959; Auerbach & Spielberger, 1972; Beck, 1960; Bohm, 1958; Fisher, 1951; Hertz, 1948; Kates & Schwartz, 1958; Klopfer et al., 1954; Levine & Spivack, 1964; Neuringer, 1962; Phillips & Smith, 1953; Piotrowski, 1957; Rapaport et al., 1946; Riessman & Miller, 1958; Schafer, 1948; Schwartz & Kates, 1957; Shapiro, 1977; Wagner & Wagner, 1978; Weiner, 1966).
2. **Subnormal number of** *FM* (Klopfer & Davidson, 1962; Levine & Spivack, 1964; Rosenzweig & Kogan, 1949).
3. ***M + FM* equal to zero or one** (Klopfer & Davidson, 1962; Levine & Spivack, 1964).
4. **Greater than normal number of inanimate movement responses** (Adams et al., 1963; Allen, 1954; Ames et al., 1952, 1974; Klopfer et al., 1954; Piotrowski, 1957).
5. **Greater than normal number of** *CF* **responses** (Bochner & Halpern, 1945; Kahn & Giffen, 1960; Schafer, 1948; Shapiro, 1960, 1977).

6. **Subnormal number of *FC* responses** (Fisher, 1951).

7. **Pure *C* responses present** (Beck, 1945; Schafer, 1948).

8. ***Csym* determinants present** (Miale, 1947).

9. **Numerous *FC* + *CF* + *C* with other determinants constructed** (Sherman, 1955).

10. **Sum *C* greater than 3** (Haworth, 1962; Hertz, 1948; Murstein, 1960; Rapaport et al., 1946).

11. **Number of *CF* greater than the number of *FC*** (Allison et al., 1968; Beck, 1945; Hertz, 1948; Munroe, 1945; Wagner & Wagner, 1978).

12. ***F*% greater than 50** (Allen, 1958; Allison et al., 1968; Ames et al., 1952, 1974; Beck, 1960; Bochner & Halpern, 1945; Consalvi & Canter, 1957; Halpern, 1953; Hertz, 1948, 1949; Hertz & Paolino, 1960; Klopfer et al., 1954; Korchin, 1960; McCue et al., 1963; Mons, 1950; Murstein, 1958; Piotrowski, 1957; Rossi & Neuman, 1961; Sarason, 1954; Schachtel, 1966; Schafer, 1954; Schwartz & Kates, 1957; Siegal et al., 1962; Singer, 1960).

13. **Sum of chromatic responses greater than 2(*Fc* + *c* + *C'*)** (Klopfer et al., 1954).

14. ***M* greater than *FM*, and *FM* equals zero or one** (Klopfer & Davidson, 1962; Rosenzweig & Kogan, 1949).

15. ***FC* + *CF* + *C* near zero** (Allen, 1954; Hertz, 1965; Klopfer et al., 1954; Palmer, 1970; Phillips & Smith, 1953).

16. ***FK* + *Fc* less than 25% *F*** (Klopfer & Davidson, 1962).

17. ***F* greater than 3(*M* + *FM*)** (Klopfer et al., 1954).

18. ***F* greater than 3(*FC* + *CF* + *C*)** (Klopfer et al., 1954).

19. ***F* greater than 3(*M* + *FM* + *FC* + *CF* + *C* + *Fc*)** (Klopfer et al., 1954).

Location and Content Indices

1. **Subnormal number of *W* locations** (Schafer, 1954).

2. **Number of *A* responses or *A*% greater than normal** (Beck, 1960; Schafer, 1954).

3. **Blood content to achromatic areas** (Phillips & Smith, 1953; Rapaport et al., 1946).

4. **Crude anatomy content emphasized** (Lindner, 1946; Pope & Scott, 1967).

5. ***M* with *A* content** (Beck, 1945, 1951).

6. **Subnormal number of content categories used** (Allen, 1958; Allison et al., 1968; Beck, 1945; Hertz, 1948, 1949; Munroe, 1945; Piotrowski, 1969; Schachtel, 1966).

7. **Colored object given to an achromatic area** (Reitzell, 1949).

Other Rorschach Indices

1. **Subnormal number of responses** (Alcock, 1963; Eichler, 1951; Fisher, 1950, 1951; Goldfried et al., 1971; Hertz, 1948, 1949; Holt, 1968; Kahn & Giffen, 1960; Miale & Harrower-Erickson, 1940; Neuringer, 1962; Olch, 1971; Phillips & Smith, 1953; Schachtel, 1966; Schafer, 1948; Sherman, 1955; Wagner, 1973; Wagner & Wagner, 1978).

2. **Vague, unelaborated language characterizes the protocol** (Levine & Spivack, 1964; Pope & Scott, 1967).

3. **Little or no expression of emotion, feelings, or mood in the protocol** (Levine & Spivack, 1964).

4. **Shock to Card II** (Alcock, 1963; Ames et al., 1959, 1971; Goldfried et al., 1971; Hertz, 1948; Klopfer et al., 1954; Miale & Harrower-Erickson, 1940; Munroe, 1945; Phillips & Smith, 1953; Piotrowski, 1957; Schachtel, 1943, 1966).

5. **Blocking to Card VIII** (Schachtel, 1966).

6. **No card turning behavior** (Smith, 1969).

7. ***W:M* shows excessive *W*** (Wagner & Wagner, 1978).

Projective Drawing Signs

1. **Random scribbled shading** (Kahn & Giffen, 1960; Schildkrout et al., 1972).

2. **Pressure unusually variable** (Urban, 1963).

3. **Marked asymmetry of human figure drawing** (Gilbert, 1969; Hammer, 1965, 1969b; Koppitz, 1966c; Machover, 1949; Mundy, 1972; Urban, 1963).

4. **Drawn person appears seductive** (McElhaney, 1969).

5. **Drawn person appears significantly younger than the subject's age** (McElhaney, 1969).

6. **Drawn person has a wide-eyed stare** (Schildkrout et al., 1972).

7. **Teeth showing in drawn person** (Buck, 1964, 1966; Halpern, 1965; Hammer, 1958, 1965; Jolles, 1971; Levy, 1950, 1958; Machover, 1949; McElhaney, 1969; Urban, 1963).

8. **Exceptionally long neck on drawn person** (Levy, 1950, 1958).

9. **Legs pressed closely together, particularly when the figure is small and shaded** (Machover, 1949; Schildkrout et al., 1972; Urban, 1963).

10. **A wide stance with lines of variable pressure** (Machover, 1949).

11. **Tree drawn with the trunk narrower at the base than elsewhere** (Koch, 1952).

Bender-Gestalt Signs
   1. **Fragmentation** (Gobetz, 1953; Hutt, 1953, 1968; Hutt & Briskin, 1960).
   2. **Dots changed to circles** (Gilbert, 1969).
   3. **Sequential reduction in size of reproductions** (Hutt & Briskin, 1960).
   4. **Exaggerated amplitude of curves on Figure 6** (Weissman & Roth, 1965).
   5. **Reduced figure size** (Hutt, 1977).

INTELLECTUALIZING OBSESSIVE-COMPULSIVE CONDITIONS
Behavioral Manifestations

Behavioral manifestations of intellectualizing obsessive-compulsive conditions, in addition to the general behavioral manifestations of neuroses, include:
   1. Ritualistic behavior such as repetitive hand washing activity or checking faucets for dripping.
   2. Excessive neatness, tidiness, and cleanliness as in ritualistically lining up all one's shoes in a straight line under the bed, repetitively shining door knobs, or scrubbing a floor repeatedly and in a stereotyped manner.
   3. Repetitive counting of items such as pencils in a desk or dishes in a cabinet.
   4. Sesquipedalianisms (in intellectualizing).
   5. Using obscure terms, frequently using them inappropriately.
   6. Regularly speaking in abstractions or theory rather than in terms of feelings and desires.

Note that most behavior directly observed as symptomatic of obsessive-compulsives tends to be compulsive in nature. The obsessions or unwanted thoughts are the ideational counterparts of compulsions or unwanted, inappropriate behavior. Obsessions are observed only through reports of the individual. However, it should be noted that some professionals feel that "the distinction between obsessions and compulsions is not particularly helpful in either research or therapy" (Ullmann & Krasner, 1975, p. 279), for both may be considered as operant behaviors. Obsessive-compulsives have been neatly and nontechnically called "checkers and cleaners" (Rachman & Hodgson, 1980). This is aptly descriptive.

Test Indices

Wechsler Signs
   1. **Unusually high Information scores** (Allison, 1978; Allison et al., 1968; Coleman & Rasof, 1963; Gilbert, 1969; Glasser & Zimmerman, 1967; Gurvitz, 1951; Holt, 1968; Mayman et al., 1951; Pope & Scott, 1967; Rapaport et al., 1945; Schafer, 1948; Wechsler, 1958).
   2. **Unusually low Comprehension scores** (Gilbert, 1969; Gurvitz, 1951; Rapaport et al., 1945; Schafer, 1948).
   3. **Comprehension scores significantly below Information scores** (Allison et al., 1968; Holt, 1968).
   4. **Unusually high Digit Span scores** (Gilbert, 1969).
   5. **Unusually high Arithmetic scores** (Rapaport et al., 1945).
   6. **Unusually high Similarities scores** (Allison et al., 1968; Gilbert, 1969; Glasser & Zimmerman, 1967; Gurvitz, 1951; Holt, 1968; Rapaport et al., 1945; Schafer, 1948; Wechsler, 1958; Zimmerman & Woo-Sam, 1973).
   7. **Unusually high Vocabulary scores** (Gilbert, 1969; Glasser & Zimmerman, 1967; Gurvitz, 1951; Holt, 1968; Mayman et al., 1951; Rapaport et al., 1945).
   8. **Unusually high Picture Completion scores** (Allison et al., 1968; Glasser & Zimmerman, 1967; Zimmerman & Woo-Sam, 1973).
   9. **Unusually low Picture Arrangement scores** (Gilbert, 1969; Gurvitz, 1951).
   10. **Unusually low Block Design scores** (Glasser & Zimmerman, 1967; Zimmerman & Woo-Sam, 1973).
   11. **VIQ significantly above PIQ** (Allison, 1978; Gurvitz, 1951; Kaufman, 1979; Maley, 1970; Mayman et al., 1951; Pope & Scott, 1967; Schafer, 1948; Wechsler, 1958).

Rorschach Signs
Indices Utilizing Determinants
   1. **Better than average quality *F* responses** (Allison et al., 1968; Beck, 1945, 1951; Holt, 1968; Korchin, 1960; Levi, 1951; Rorschach, 1921/1951).
   2. **Greater than normal number of inanimate movement responses** (Kates, 1950).
   3. ***M* determinants with *Hd* content** (Phillips & Smith, 1953).
   4. **Greater than normal number of *FC* responses** (Haworth, 1962; Kates, 1950; Rapaport et al., 1946; Shapiro, 1960).
   5. ***FC* + *CF* + *C* approximately zero** (Alcock, 1963; Shatin, 1952; Sherman, 1955).
   6. **Sum *C* greater than 3** (Haworth, 1962; Hertz, 1948; Murstein, 1960; Rapaport et al., 1946).
   7. **Superior quality *FC* responses with *dr* locations** (Schafer, 1954).
   8. **Subnormal number of pair and reflection responses** (Exner, 1978).
   9. ***F/C* responses are present** (Shapiro, 1977).

Indices Utilizing Locations

1. ***Dd*** **locations used in greater than normal number** (Allen, 1954; Allison et al., 1968; Ames et al., 1952, 1974; Beck, 1945, 1978; Bochner & Halpern, 1945; Bohm, 1958; Exner, 1974; Fisher, 1950; Goldfarb, 1943; Goldfried et al., 1971; Gurvitz, 1951; Hertz, 1948; Holt, 1968; Kahn & Giffen, 1960; Klopfer et al., 1954; Levi, 1965; Piotrowski, 1957; Sarason, 1954; Weiner, 1977).

2. ***dd*** **locations used in greater than normal number** (Alcock, 1963; Beck, 1945; Ferguson, 1952; Goldfarb, 1943; Klopfer & Davidson, 1962; Piotrowski, 1957; Rosenzweig & Kogan, 1949).

3. ***dr*** **locations used in greater than normal number** (Alcock, 1963; Allison et al., 1968; Holt, 1968; Kates, 1950; Klopfer et al., 1954; Rapaport et al., 1946; Rosenzweig & Kogan, 1949; Schafer, 1948, 1954).

4. ***de*** **locations used in greater than normal number** (Bochner & Halpern, 1945; Holt, 1968; Phillips & Smith, 1953; Schafer, 1954).

5. ***Dd*** **+** ***S*** **locations used in greater than normal number** (Alcock, 1963).

6. ***do*** **responses present** (Holt, 1968; Piotrowski, 1957).

7. ***S*** **locations used in greater than normal number** (DeKoninck & Crabbe-Decleve, 1971).

8. ***DdS*** **with** ***dr*** **locations used in greater than normal number** (Alcock, 1963).

9. ***d*** **locations used in greater than normal number** (Gurvitz, 1951; Halpern, 1953; Klopfer & Davidson, 1962; Levitt & Truumaa, 1972; Piotrowski, 1957; Schafer, 1954).

10. ***W–*** **and** ***Wv*** **responses given** (Allen, 1954; Bochner & Halpern, 1945; Gurvitz, 1951; Klopfer & Davidson, 1962; Sarason, 1954; Schafer, 1954).

11. ***W,S*** **and** ***D,S*** **locations used frequently** (Fonda, 1977).

Indices Utilizing Content Categories

1. ***Hd*** **content used in greater than normal number** (Klopfer & Davidson, 1962; Molish, 1967; Phillips & Smith, 1953).

2. **Animal content used in greater than normal number** (Goldfried et al., 1971; Kahn & Giffen, 1960; Miale & Harrower-Erickson, 1940; Schafer, 1948).

3. ***H*** **+** ***A*** **less than (***Hd*** **+** ***Ad***) **times two** (Alcock, 1963; Allison et al., 1968; Klopfer & Davidson, 1962; Phillips & Smith, 1953; Schafer, 1948).

4. **Anal content emphasized** (Brar, 1970; Goldfried et al., 1971; Lindner, 1946, 1947, 1950; Phillips & Smith, 1953; Piotrowski, 1957; Schafer, 1948, 1954).

5. **Unusually high** ***Ad%*** (Goldfried et al., 1971; Kahn & Giffen, 1960; Miale & Harrower-Erickson, 1940; Schafer, 1948).

6. **Unusually large number of anatomy responses** (Exner, 1974).

Other Rorschach Indices

1. **An abnormally large number of responses** (Alcock, 1963; Allen, 1954; Beck, 1951; Bochner & Halpern, 1945; Halpern, 1960; Holt, 1968; Kahn & Giffen, 1960; Kates, 1950; Pope & Scott, 1967; Sherman, 1955).

2. **Fabulized combinations noted where content is part one thing and part another** (Rapaport et al., 1946; Schafer, 1948).

3. **Criticizing the Rorschach plates** (Schafer, 1948).

4. **Symmetry comments emphasized** (Beck, 1978).

Projective Drawing Signs

Graphological and General Indices

1. **Very light pressure** (Hammer, 1954c, 1958; Handler & Reyher, 1966; Jolles, 1971; Machover, 1955; Precker, 1950; Urban, 1963).

2. **Excessive erasing** (Kahn & Giffen, 1960; Machover, 1949; Reynolds, 1978; Urban, 1963).

3. **Placement on the right side of the page** (Buck, 1948, 1950, 1964; Hammer, 1958; Jolles, 1971; Jolles & Beck, 1953a).

4. **Very small drawings** (Brick, 1944).

5. **Excessive detailing** (Buck, 1948, 1964, 1966; Deabler, 1969; Hammer, 1954c, 1958, 1965, 1969a, 1969b; Jacks, 1969; Kahn & Giffen, 1960; Levy, 1958; Machover, 1949; McElhaney, 1969; Reynolds, 1978).

6. **Extreme bilateral symmetry** (Hammer, 1958; Machover, 1949, 1951; Urban, 1963).

Draw-A-Person/Human Figure Drawing Indices

1. **Unusually small head** (Buck, 1964, 1966; Gilbert, 1969; Jolles, 1971; Machover, 1949; Urban, 1963).

2. **Tiny mouths** (Urban, 1963).

3. **Detailing or emphasizing of joints of fingers and fingernails** (Levy, 1950, 1958; Machover, 1949; Urban, 1963).

4. **Excessive detailing of feet** (Buck, 1966; Jolles, 1971; Urban, 1963).

5. **Arms stiff at the sides of the body** (Buck, 1964; Hammer, 1954c; Jacks, 1969; Jolles, 1971; Machover, 1949; Schildkrout et al., 1972).

6. **Monotonously striped clothing** (Schildkrout et al., 1972).

7. **Buttons drawn on cuffs** (Levy, 1958; Machover, 1949; Urban, 1963).

House and Tree Drawing Indices
1. **Transparent walls** (Buck, 1948; Jolles, 1971).
2. **Branches drawn turning inward, not outward** (Buck, 1964, 1966; Hammer, 1958).
3. **Bark meticulously drawn** (Jolles, 1971).
4. **Leaves meticulously drawn in two dimensions** (Buck, 1964, 1966; Jolles, 1971).
5. **Numerous leaves not attached to branches** (Levine & Sapolsky, 1969).
6. **An excessive number of leaves drawn** (Levine & Sapolsky, 1969).
7. **Shadows cast by the tree** (Jolles, 1971).

Bender-Gestalt Signs
1. **Numbering and boxing-off of figures** (Billingslea, 1948; DeCato & Wicks, 1976; Gilbert, 1969; Gobetz, 1953; Lerner, 1972; Woltmann, 1950).
2. **Perseverations** (Gobetz, 1953; Hutt & Briskin, 1960).
3. **More than three or four minutes used on each design** (Gilbert, 1969).
4. **Rigidly methodical arrangements** (Billingslea, 1948; Halpern, 1951; Hutt, 1953, 1968; Hutt & Briskin, 1960; Woltmann, 1950).
5. **Emphasizing pairing of dots on Figure 1** (Lerner, 1972).
6. **General difficulty with Figure 1** (Hutt & Briskin, 1960).
7. **Counting dots repeatedly on Figure 5 and losing the gestalt by concentrating on accurate dot reproduction** (Gobetz, 1953; Hutt & Briskin, 1960; Lerner, 1972; Story, 1960; Weissman & Roth, 1965).
8. **Sketching and then marking dots on Figure 5** (Lerner, 1972).
9. **On Figure 6, a reduction in size or curvature** (Suczek & Klopfer, 1952; Weissman & Roth, 1965).
10. **General difficulty with, or spending considerable time on, Figure 1** (Hutt, 1977; Hutt & Briskin, 1960).

Contraindication

1. **Rejections or failures on the Rorschach** (Holt, 1968).

FEARS AND PHOBIAS

There is a dimension of emotional behaviors, characterized by an unpleasant, frightening feeling that is accompanied by sympathetic nervous system activity and sundry postural and motor activities, that extends from fear to phobia (cf. English & English, 1958; Hinsie & Campbell, 1970; Rycroft, 1973; Warren, 1934). Fear may be considered as an essentially normal response to a dangerous stimulus or situation. A fright reaction to a mad dog or to the approach of a tornado is appropriate and normal.

A phobia, on the other hand, is an intense fear which is to some extent incapacitating and irrational. The expression "morbid dread" may not be too vivid a description of the phobic experience. For a frightened reaction to be considered phobic, the response must be inappropriate or disproportionate to the stimulus. Fears, then, are sometimes normal, whereas phobias are not. Among the classical forms of neuroses, phobias were considered one of the symptoms of psychasthenia. Current thought holds that phobias may be found in any neurosis and occasionally are found in individuals who are otherwise normal. The new diagnostic manual (DSM-III) of the American Psychiatric Association (1980) notes that features associated with phobias include rituals and compulsions as with the old nosological entity *psychasthenia*, though this term is eschewed in that manual.

The variety of specific phobias is, for practical purposes, uncountable. Hall (1914) listed 135 phobias. Numberous additional phobias have appeared in the literature since that time.

DSM-III divides all phobic disorders into three types: Agoraphobia, Social Phobia, and Simple Phobia. *Agoraphobia*, in the DSM-III context, refers to an irrational dread of open, public places, but also includes ochlophobia (a fear of crowds) and claustrophobia (fear of enclosed places such as tunnels and elevators). *Social phobia* denotes the persistent, irrational fear of being "exposed to scrutiny by others." An exaggerated, durable fear of crowds and of being humiliated or embarrassed is associated with social phobia. The most frequently encountered example of this is a type of lalophobia, fear of speaking or performing in public. *Simple phobia* is the "everything else" category. "Thus, this is a residual category of Phobic Disorders . . . and . . . are sometimes referred to as 'specific' phobias" (American Psychiatric Association, 1980, pp. 228-229). Mentioned as examples of simple phobias are acrophobia and claustrophobia, which also fits into the broad definition in DSM-III of agoraphobia. This classification scheme may be considered exhaustive but the categories certainly are not mutually exclusive.

Behavioral Manifestations

Behavioral manifestations of phobias include:
1. Becoming immobilized, freezing in one's tracks.
2. Flight or running pell-mell from the phobic stimulus.
3. Trembling.

4. Dizziness or fainting.
5. Profuse perspiring.
6. Flushing.

Most of the autonomic responses observed in anxiety attacks may also be manifested here. For some, "The primary distinction between anxiety reactions and phobic reactions is that the latter are associated with specific situations or objects" (Martin, 1977, p. 148). Inasmuch as behavioral expressions of the two conditions are so similar, appropriate reference may be made to the manifestations of anxiety noted previously in this chapter.

Test Indices

Wechsler Signs
1. **Unusually low Similarities scores** (Glasser & Zimmerman, 1967).

Rorschach Signs

Determinant, Location, and Content Indices
1. **Greater than normal number of achromatic responses** (Ames et al., 1952, 1974; Phillips & Smith, 1953; Piotrowski, 1957; Wagner, 1971).
2. **Surface shading plus achromatic responses greater than twice the number of chromatic—$Fc + c + C'$ greater than $2(FC + CF + C)$** (Arnaud, 1959; Klopfer et al., 1954).
3. **Greater than normal number of *de* responses** (Alcock, 1963; Allen, 1954, 1958; Klopfer & Davidson, 1962).
4. ***Hd* content of a human limb** (Phillips & Smith, 1953).
5. **Spider content** (Pope & Scott, 1967).
6. **Blood content** (Brar, 1970; Elizur, 1949; Haworth, 1962; Lindner, 1946; Phillips & Smith, 1953).
7. **Crude anatomy content** (Lindner, 1946; Pope & Scott, 1967).
8. **Mountain and hilly landscape content emphasized** (Rychlak, 1959).
9. **Ugly, weird, loathsome, huge, menacing, sinister, frightful content emphasized** (Aronow & Reznikoff, 1976).
10. **Subnormal number of pair and reflection responses** (Exner, 1978).
11. **Greater than normal number of (H) responses** (Molish, 1967).

Other Rorschach Indices
1. **Greater than normal number of Popular responses** (Allen, 1954; Ames et al., 1959, 1971; Beck, 1945; Klopfer et al., 1954; Levitt & Truumaa, 1972; Murstein, 1958; Piotrowski, 1957; Rapaport et al., 1946; Schafer, 1948).

2. **Shock to Card II** (Phillips & Smith, 1953).
3. **Shock to Card IV** (Ames et al., 1971; Bohm, 1960; Goldfried et al., 1971; Schachtel, 1966).
4. **Shock to Card VI** (Goldfried et al., 1971; Klopfer et al., 1954; Phillips & Smith, 1953; Piotrowski, 1957).

Projective Drawing Signs
1. **Unusually light pressure** (Buck, 1969; DiLeo, 1970, 1973; Hammer, 1954c, 1968; Jolles, 1971; Kadis, 1950; Reynolds, 1978; Rosenzweig & Kogan, 1949; Machover, 1949; Urban, 1963).
2. **Excessive details** (Hammer, 1965, 1969b).
3. **Belts on human figure drawings that are elaborate or emphasized** (Buck, 1964, 1966; Jolles, 1971; Machover, 1949; Urban, 1963).
4. **Horizontal line emphasis** (Alschuler & Hattwick, 1947; Levy, 1950, 1958).
5. **Trees drawn leaning significantly** (Buck, 1964; Jolles, 1971; Koch, 1952).
6. **Tall, narrow branches reaching up, not out** (Jolles, 1971).

Bender-Gestalt Signs
1. **Crowded, compressed, cohesive arrangements** (Brown, 1965; Clawson, 1959, 1962; Haworth & Rabin, 1960; Hutt, 1953, 1977; Hutt & Briskin, 1960; Woltmann, 1950).
2. **Overlapping and crossing difficulty** (Hutt, 1953, 1977; Hutt & Gibby, 1970).
3. **Upper left-hand corner placement** (Hutt, 1953).
4. **Unusually small reproductions** (Hutt, 1977).
5. **On Figure 3, reduced size, increased right-hand angle, and preoccupation with detail rather than form** (Suczek & Klopfer, 1952).
6. **Dots on Figure 5 converge** (Lerner, 1972; Weissman & Roth, 1965).
7. **On Figure 6, two more or less tangential "U" curves are substituted for the crossing** (Hutt & Briskin, 1960).

Contraindication

1. **Better than average quality F responses on the Rorschach** (Goldman, 1960).

CHAPTER 4
PSYCHOSES AND RELATED PHENOMENA

REALITY TIES

Good reality ties, from our point of view, anchor the healthy end of the spectrum of reality ties though this is short of "perfect reality ties." The discussion of normality (see Chapter 2) pointed out the distinction between normality and perfection. Individuals may function in a "better than average" or "very good" manner though they are by no means perfect. The other end of this spectrum is anchored, for us, by the poor reality ties observed in psychotics. As Coleman (1972) pointed out, "The schizophrenic tends to withdraw from reality into a world of fantasy and private experience" (p. 272). While their ties with reality may be exceedingly strained, rarely if ever do they reach the point of zero reality contact. In this volume, weak and loose reality ties refer to conditions that exist between good and poor reality ties.

Two points need to be made here. First, "Bizarre behavior [as associated with poor reality ties] is typically episodic" (Coleman, 1972, p. 273). Most if not all psychotics still have some intermittent contact with reality. The other point goes beyond noting that normals are not perfectly realistic in their perceptions and behavior. Reality, in the strict sense, may be unknowable. Psychologists and people in general deal with a consensually agreed upon view of reality, which in fact is all we really know. A philosophical consideration of the difference between Reality and The Way Things Seem is obviously beyond the scope of this work.

Behavioral Manifestations

Manifestations of *good reality ties* include acts which are understandable, purposeful, and appropriate. Detailing this kind of behavior becomes as awesome as detailing normal behavior. For some additional considerations, refer to the somewhat more detailed discussion of normal behavior in Chapter 2.

Manifestations of *weak or loose reality ties* include acts which are only relatively incredible, though not thoroughly preposterous. Behavior describable as peculiar and nonsensical tends to fall into this category.

Manifestations of *poor reality ties* include most of the bizarre acts of psychotics and some others under the influence of drugs. This type of behavior is quite absurd or preposterous, and with minimal, if any, immediately apparent logical explanation. At times, through careful analytic procedures, a devious explanation or tortuous logic may be uncovered even for this bizarre behavior.

Test Indices of Good Reality Ties

Rorschach Signs

1. **Greater than average number of M** (Adams et al., 1963; Allen, 1954, 1958; Barrell, 1953; Cooper & Caston, 1970; Dana, 1968; Davids & Talmadge, 1964; Goldfried et al., 1971; Kaden & Lipton, 1960; Kahn, 1967; Kates & Schwartz, 1958; King, 1958, 1960; Klopfer & Davidson, 1962; Kurz, 1963; Levine et al., 1957; Levitt & Truumaa, 1972; Nickerson, 1969; Phillips & Smith, 1953; Piotrowski, 1937a, 1957, 1960, 1969; Piotrowski & Bricklin, 1961; Schumer cited in Sarason, 1954; Singer, 1955, 1960; Singer et al., 1956; Singer & Herman, 1954; Singer & Sugarman, 1955; Spivack et al., 1959; Wagner, 1971).
2. **Average number of M** (Adams et al., 1963; Klopfer & Davidson, 1962; Phillips & Smith, 1953; Piotrowski, 1957).
3. **Average or better quality of M responses** (Klopfer et al., 1954).
4. **Better than average quality F responses** (Adams et al., 1963; Beck, 1945, 1968; Beck et al., 1961; Bohm, 1958; Goldman, 1960; Halpern, 1953; Hertz, 1960; Kodman & Waters, 1961; Korchin, 1960; Lerner & Shanan, 1972; Levitt & Truumaa, 1972; Mayman, 1970; Piotrowski, 1957; Rickers-Ovsiankina, 1960; Sarason, 1954; Schachtel, 1966; Schafer, 1954; Williams, 1947).
5. **Normal number of P responses** (Klopfer & Davidson, 1962; Schafer, 1954).

Test Indices of Weak or Loose Reality Ties

Rorschach Signs

1. **Subnormal quality inanimate movement responses** (Allen, 1954).
2. **Presence of do responses** (Holt, 1968; Klopfer et al., 1954).
3. **$Dd + S$ present in greater than normal number** (Fonda, 1960; Klopfer et al., 1954; Neuringer, 1962).
4. **Subnormal number of P responses** (Allen, 1954; Ames et al., 1959, 1971; Beck, 1960; Klopfer & Davidson, 1962; Rapaport et al., 1946; Schwartz & Giacoman, 1972).
5. **Low $D\%$, poor form level with few P responses** (Klopfer et al., 1954).
6. **Generally poor form level** (Beck & Molish, 1967).

Projective Drawing Signs

1. **Tiptoe stance on drawing of Person** (Hammer, 1954c; Jolles, 1971; Urban, 1963).
2. **Vertical dimension of H-T-P House drawing strongly overemphasized** (Buck, 1964; Jolles, 1971).
3. **House drawing sitting on a spontaneously drawn cloud-like ground line** (Hammer, 1969a).
4. **Walls to House drawing unconnected with a base line** (Jolles, 1971).
5. **H-T-P Tree drawn with talon-like roots** (Jolles, 1971).

Test Indices of Poor Reality Ties

Rorschach Signs

1. **Poor quality *F* responses predominate** (Allen, 1954; Beck, 1944, 1945, 1951, 1968; Berkowitz & Levine, 1953; Bohm, 1958; Gottlieb & Parsons, 1960; Hertz & Paolino, 1960; Holt, 1968; Kahn & Giffen, 1960; Kalinowsky & Hoch, 1961; Kataguchi, 1959; Korchin, 1960; Neiger, Slemon, & Quirk, 1962; Phillips & Smith, 1953; Piotrowski, 1957; Piotrowski & Berg, 1955; Piotrowski & Bricklin, 1961; Piotrowski & Lewis, 1950; Rapaport et al., 1946; Schafer, 1948, 1954, 1960; Weiner, 1961b; Wolman, 1972).
2. **_F%_ greater than 80** (Klopfer & Davidson, 1962).
3. **_M-_ responses present** (Beck, 1951; Gurvitz, 1951; Hertz & Paolino, 1960; Klopfer et al., 1954; Phillips & Smith, 1953; Schachtel, 1966).
4. **_FM-_ responses present** (Hertz & Paolino, 1960).
5. **_DW_ responses present** (Allen, 1954; Ames et al., 1952, 1974; Bochner & Halpern, 1945; Klopfer & Davidson, 1962; Piotrowski, 1957).
6. **_Ad_ content present in greater than normal number** (Allen, 1954; Bohm, 1958).
7. **_O-_ responses present** (Alcock, 1963; Allen, 1954, 1958; Bochner & Halpern, 1945; Bohm, 1958; Hertz & Paolino, 1960; Kalinowski & Hoch, 1961; Klopfer et al., 1954; Miale, 1947; Pierce, Cooke, & Frahm, 1973; Quirk, Quarrington, Neiger, & Slemon, 1962; Rapaport et al., 1946; Rorschach, 1921/1951).
8. **Confabulations, abnormal content combinations** (Klopfer et al., 1954; Rapaport et al., 1946).

Projective Drawing Signs

1. **Gross distortions in drawings** (Burton & Sjoberg, 1964; Hozier, 1959; Jacks, 1969; Kahn & Giffen, 1960; McElhaney, 1969).
2. **Any unrealistic transparency present** (Ogdon, 1975; Reynolds, 1978).

3. **H-T-P House drawing with chimney smoke blowing both to left and to right** (Buck, 1964; Hammer, 1954c, 1969a; Jolles, 1971).
4. **Absence of walls in House drawing** (Hammer, 1954c; Jolles, 1971).
5. **Transparent walls in House drawing** (Buck, 1948, 1964; Deabler, 1969; Hammer, 1958; Jolles, 1971; Levine & Sapolsky, 1969).
6. **H-T-P Tree drawing with transparent roots, or trunks seen through the groundline** (Buck, 1948, 1964, 1966).
7. **Thin roots on Tree drawing making tenuous contact with the ground** (Hammer, 1954c; Jolles, 1971; Mursell, 1969).
8. **Tree drawn with dead roots** (Buck, 1964; Jolles, 1971).

Bender-Gestalt Signs

1. **Marked perseverations** (Hutt, 1953, 1968; Hutt & Briskin, 1960).
2. **Spontaneous elaborations manifested** (Hutt, 1978).
3. **Great variability in the size of the reproductions** (DeCato & Wicks, 1976).

PSYCHOSES: GENERAL CONSIDERATIONS

Behavioral Manifestations

Behavior of psychotics is in many respects further from normal than is the behavior of individuals in any other section of this volume. Psychoses are most serious psychological disorders involving severe personality disorganization and loss of contact with reality.

Four characteristics tend to set psychotics apart. Hallucinatory behavior is one. False sensory experiences of seeing, hearing, feeling, and to a lesser extent smelling or tasting things for which there is no adequate external stimulus, mark a psychotic.

Delusions are a second characteristic. These include false ideas of reference which are not corrected when information is available to indicate the ideas are erroneous. Among other more commonly encountered delusions are false ideas of grandeur, unrealistic feelings of power and control that may be manifested, as well as feelings of persecution or that one's behavior is being controlled by others.

Disorientation in any of the three major spheres of person, place, or time also suggests psychosis. Individuals who do not know who they are, or perhaps think they are someone else such as Napoleon, George Washington, etc., are disoriented as to person. The belief that one is living in another time, either in the past or future, marks disorientation as to time. Individuals who do not know where they are, or think they are somewhere they are not, are not properly oriented in place.

The fourth characteristic of psychotic behavior is bizarre activity. The psychotic may display wildly improbable behavior. This activity may be dangerous to the patient or others, or it may be relatively innocuous. Sitting on a chair, fully clothed, in a shower with the water running exemplifies innocuous bizarre behavior.

Presence of hallucinations, delusions, disorientation or bizarre behavior always raises the probability of a psychotic condition. These characterize both organic and functional psychoses. Care must be taken, however, to rule out transient effects of drugs which sometimes mimic the more durable symptomatology of psychoses.

Test Indices

Wechsler Signs

1. **Verbal IQ significantly greater than Performance IQ** (Garfield, 1949; Gilbert, 1969; Goldfarb, 1961; Guertin et al., 1966; Gurvitz, 1951; Kahn & Giffen, 1960; Pope & Scott, 1967; Rabin, 1942; Sinnett & Mayman, 1960; Wechsler, 1958).

2. **Several early, easy Information items missed and more difficult items passed** (Holt, 1968; Rapaport et al., 1945).

3. **Significantly more Digits Forward given correctly than Digits Backward** (Holt, 1968).

4. **Unusually low Arithmetic score, especially when combined with unusually low Comprehension or Picture Arrangement score** (Allison, 1978; Glasser & Zimmerman, 1967; Gurvitz, 1951; Holt, 1968; Kahn & Giffen, 1960; Magaret, 1942; Rapaport et al., 1945; Schafer, 1948).

5. **Very wide subtest scatter** (Allison, 1978; Allison et al., 1968; Rapaport et al., 1945).

Rorschach Signs

Determinant Indices

1. **Poor quality F responses** (Allen, 1954; Beck, 1944, 1945, 1951, 1968; Berkowitz & Levine, 1953; Bohm, 1958; Gottlieb & Parsons, 1960; Harrow, Quinlan, Wollington, & Pickett, 1976; Hertz & Paolino, 1960; Holt, 1968; Kahn & Giffen, 1960; Kalinowsky & Hoch, 1961; Kataguchi, 1959; Korchin, 1960; Neiger et al., 1962; Phillips & Smith, 1953; Piotrowski, 1957; Piotrowski & Berg, 1955; Piotrowski & Bricklin, 1961; Piotrowski & Lewis, 1950; Rapaport et al., 1946; Schafer, 1948, 1954, 1960; Weiner, 1961b; Wolman, 1972).

2. **Erratic quality of form level** (Allen, 1954; Kahn & Giffen, 1960).

3. **F% greater than 50** (Adams et al., 1963; Allen, 1954; Beck, 1960; Klopfer et al., 1954; Rapaport et al., 1946; Schafer, 1948; Vinson, 1960).

4. **Subnormal number of M** (Alcock, 1963; Bohm, 1958; Evans & Marmorston, 1963; Goldfried et al., 1971; Harrower-Erickson, 1941; Hughes, 1948, 1950; Kahn & Giffen, 1960; Kisker, 1944; Klopfer et al., 1954; Neiger et al., 1962; Oberholzer cited in Kisker, 1944; Phillips & Smith, 1953; Piotrowski, 1937b, 1960).

5. **Subnormal quality M responses** (Beck, 1951; Blatt, Brenneis, Shimek, & Glick, 1976; Exner, 1974; Phillips & Smith, 1953; Schafer, 1948).

6. **M + FM equal to or less than one** (Klopfer & Davidson, 1962).

7. **Subnormal number or an absence of Fc** (Rapaport et al., 1946).

8. **FC + CF + C is approximately zero** (Bochner & Halpern, 1945; Bohm, 1958; Hertz, 1948, 1949; Piotrowski & Levine, 1959; Rapaport et al., 1946; Rorschach, 1921/1951; Schafer, 1960; Shapiro, 1960).

Location and Content Indices

1. **DW responses present** (Alcock, 1963; Beck, 1945; Bochner & Halpern, 1945; Friedman, 1953; Goldfried et al., 1971; Holt, 1968; Klopfer et al., 1954; Phillips & Smith, 1953; Piotrowski, 1957; Rapaport et al., 1946; Rorschach, 1921/1951; Schafer, 1948; Thiesen, 1952; Vinson, 1960; Watkins & Stauffacher, 1952).

2. **Space response to Card VIII** (Lindner, 1950).

3. **Alphabet, numbers, punctuation or geometric content** (Bohm, 1958; Brar, 1970; Klopfer & Davidson, 1962; Orme, 1963; Phillips & Smith, 1953; Piotrowski, 1957; Schafer, 1948, 1954).

4. **Vague W locations with anatomy content** (Sherman, 1955).

5. **Malevolent H content** (Blatt et al., 1976; Ritzler, Zambianco, Harder, & Kaskey, 1980).

6. **Subnormal quality of H responses** (Blatt et al., 1976).

7. **Unusually large number of (H) or Hd- responses** (Blatt et al., 1976).

Other Rorschach Indices

1. **O- responses present** (Alcock, 1963; Allen, 1954, 1958; Bochner & Halpern, 1945; Bohm, 1958; Hertz & Paolino, 1960; Kalinowski & Hoch, 1961; Klopfer et al., 1954; Miale, 1947; Pierce et al., 1973; Quirk et al., 1962; Rapaport et al., 1946; Rorschach, 1921/1951).

2. **Subnormal number of _P_** (Alcock, 1963; Allen, 1954; Beck, 1945; Berkowitz & Levine, 1953; Bochner & Halpern, 1945; Bohm, 1958; Goldfried et al., 1971; Kataguchi, 1959; Knopf, 1956, 1965; Pierce et al., 1973; Schafer, 1948, 1960; Thiesen, 1952; Vinson, 1960).

3. **Subnormal number of responses** (Alcock, 1963; Allen, 1954; Ames, Learned, Metraux, & Walker, 1954; Ames, Metraux, Rodell, & Walker, 1973; Bradway & Heisler, 1953; Evans & Marmorston, 1963; Goldfried et al., 1971; Harrower-Erickson, 1941; Hertz & Loehrke, 1954; Hughes, 1948, 1950; Kahn & Giffen, 1960; Kisker, 1944; Kral & Dorken, 1953; Neiger et al., 1962; Piotrowski, 1937b, 1957).

4. **Confabulations, abnormal content combinations, or content changes during performance** (Allen, 1958; Klopfer et al., 1954; Quirk et al., 1962; Rapaport et al., 1946).

5. **Contaminations, abnormal thought combinations present** (Alcock, 1963; Allen, 1958; Allison, 1978; Beck, 1945; Carlson et al., 1973; Friedman, 1952, 1953; Goldfried et al., 1971; Halpern, 1953; Hertz, 1960; Hertz & Paolino, 1960; Kelley & Klopfer, 1939; Klopfer et al., 1954; Miale, 1947; Phillips & Smith, 1953; Piotrowski, 1957, 1969; Pope & Scott, 1967; Quirk et al., 1962; Rapaport et al., 1946; Schafer, 1948; Watkins & Stauffacher, 1952).

6. **Edging behavior** (Allen, 1954; Baker, 1956; Beck, 1945; Klopfer et al., 1954; Phillips & Smith, 1953).

7. **Shock to Card IV** (Berkowitz & Levine, 1953; Goldfried et al., 1971; Piotrowski, 1957; Piotrowski & Berg, 1955; Piotrowski & Lewis, 1950).

8. **Shock to Card V** (Bohm, 1958; Brown, 1953; Klopfer et al., 1954; McCully, 1971; Piotrowski, 1957).

9. **Shock to Card VI** (Goldfried et al., 1971; Klopfer et al., 1954; Phillips & Smith, 1953; Piotrowski, 1957).

10. **Confused sequences, less than three cards treated systematically** (Allen, 1954).

Projective Drawing Signs
Graphological and General Indices

1. **Tremulous, shaky, uncoordinated lines** (McElhaney, 1969).

2. **Gross distortions present** (Burton & Sjoberg, 1964; Hozier, 1959; Jacks, 1969; Kahn & Giffen, 1960; McElhaney, 1969).

3. **Bizarre details present** (Buck, 1964, 1966; Kahn & Giffen, 1960; Koppitz, 1960; McElhaney, 1969; Mursell, 1969).

4. **Labeling of details** (McElhaney, 1969).

Draw-A-Person/Human Figure Drawing Indices

1. **Unusually large head** (McElhaney, 1969).

2. **Irregular contour of head** (Machover, 1949).

3. **Confusion of profile and full face** (Gilbert, 1969; Kahn & Giffen, 1960; Machover, 1949; Urban, 1963).

4. **Dehumanized human figure as boxy, robot-, manikin-, or monster-like, or with a geometric shape** (Chase, 1941; McElhaney, 1969; Reynolds, 1978).

5. **Clear indications of internal organs** (Buck, 1966; Kahn & Giffen, 1960; Levy, 1950, 1958; Machover, 1949, 1951; McElhaney, 1969; Reynolds, 1978; Urban, 1963).

6. **Grossly disorganized or fragmented figures** (Kahn & Giffen, 1960; Koppitz, 1960, 1968; McElhaney, 1969; Modell, 1951; Reynolds, 1978; Reznikoff & Tomblen, 1956; Schildkrout et al., 1972; Small, 1973).

7. **Facial features omitted** (Gurvitz, 1951; McElhaney, 1969).

8. **Ears unusually large or strongly reinforced** (Buck, 1964; Deabler, 1969; Hammer, 1954c, 1968, 1978; Jolles, 1971; Levy, 1950, 1958; Machover, 1949; Mursell, 1969; Schildkrout et al., 1972; Urban, 1963).

9. **Ears omitted** (Buck, 1966; Deabler, 1969; DiLeo, 1973; Jolles, 1971).

10. **Dark dots drawn in ear area** (Schildkrout et al., 1972).

11. **Eyes omitted** (Buck, 1964; Jolles, 1969, 1971).

12. **Pupil omitted from only one eye** (McElhaney, 1969).

13. **Transparent clothing** (Holzberg & Wexler, 1950; Hozier, 1959; Machover, 1949; McElhaney, 1969).

H-T-P House and Tree Drawing Indices

1. **Double perspective with both end walls exaggerated** (Buck, 1948; Deabler, 1969; Hammer, 1954c; Jolles, 1971).

2. **Transparent walls on House drawing** (Buck, 1948, 1964; Deabler, 1969; Hammer, 1958; Jolles, 1971; Levine & Sapolsky, 1969).

3. **House drawn only as a roof (not as an A-frame dwelling)** (Buck, 1964; Deabler, 1969; Hammer, 1954c, 1958).

4. **Smoke from chimney blowing both to left and to right** (Buck, 1964; Hammer, 1954c, 1969a; Jolles, 1971).
5. **Doors omitted from House drawing** (Beck, 1955; Buck, 1948; Deabler, 1969; Jolles, 1971).
6. **Windows omitted** (Deabler, 1969).
7. **Shades extending outside the windows** (Hammer, 1969a).
8. **Split Tree drawing: two one-dimensional trees side by side, each with an independent branch structure** (Buck, 1948; Deabler, 1969; Hammer, 1954c, 1958; Jacks, 1969; Jolles, 1971; Koch, 1952; Landisberg, 1958; Levine & Sapolsky, 1969).
9. **Branch structure of Tree drawing is very similar to the root structure** (Hammer, 1969a).

Bender-Gestalt Signs
Unusual Reproduction Modes
1. **Fragmentation** (Allen, 1958; Bender, 1938; Clawson, 1962; Gilbert, 1969; Guertin, 1954a; Halpern, 1951; Hutt, 1953, 1968, 1977, 1978; Hutt & Briskin, 1960; Hutt & Gibby, 1970; Woltmann, 1950).
2. **Overlapping and crossing difficulty** (Bender, 1938; Gilbert, 1969; Goldberg, 1956-57; Halpern, 1951; Hutt, 1977; Hutt & Gibby, 1970; Koppitz, 1958).
3. **Rotations** (Allen, 1958; Bender, 1956; DeCato & Wicks, 1976; Gilbert, 1969; Goldberg, 1956-57; Griffith & Taylor, 1960; Guertin, 1952; Halpern, 1951; Hutt, 1953, 1968, 1977; Hutt & Briskin, 1960; Hutt & Gibby, 1970; Kahn & Giffen, 1960; Woltmann, 1950).
4. **Spontaneous elaborations, embellishments, and doodling** (Bender, 1938; Gilbert, 1969; Hutt, 1953, 1977; Hutt & Briskin, 1960; Hutt & Gibby, 1970; Woltmann, 1950).
5. **Excessive workover** (Pascal & Suttell, 1951; Woltmann, 1950).
6. **Severe perseveration** (Hutt, 1977).
7. **Closure difficulty manifested** (Hutt, 1977).
8. **Regression including retrogression and simplification** (Hutt, 1977).
9. **Dots substituted for circles** (Hutt, 1977).

Unusual Arrangements and Specific Figure Treatment
1. **Collision arrangement** (Clawson, 1962; DeCato & Wicks, 1976; Guertin, 1954c; Halpern, 1951; Hutt, 1953, 1968, 1977; Hutt & Briskin, 1960; Hutt & Gibby, 1970).
2. **Confused or chaotic arrangement** (Bender, 1938; Goldberg, 1956-57; Guertin, 1954c; Halpern, 1951; Hutt, 1953, 1968; Hutt & Briskin, 1960).
3. **Crowded, compressed, or cohesive arrangements** (Bender, 1938; Gilbert, 1969; Goldberg, 1956-57; Guertin, 1955; Halpern, 1951; Hutt, 1968).
4. **An expanded, enormous reproduction of Figure 1** (Lerner, 1972).
5. **On Figure 2 dots or lines substituted for circles** (Hutt, 1968).
6. **Sequentially increasing distortions of the figures** (DeCato & Wicks, 1976).
7. **Figure A placed in a lower corner** (Hutt, 1977).

Contraindications
1. **Rorschach *M* responses with abstract content** (Phillips & Smith, 1953).
2. **Unusually large number of inanimate movement responses on the Rorschach** (Klopfer et al., 1956).
3. **Number of Rorschach responses greater than 40 with number of Popular responses greater than 7** (Bradway & Heisler, 1953).
4. **Greater than average number of Popular responses on the Rorschach** (Beck, 1960; Berkowitz & Levine, 1953; Bradway & Heisler, 1953; Hertz, 1948; Mundy, 1972; Piotrowski, 1957; Rapaport et al., 1946).
5. **Better than average quality *F* responses** (Adams et al., 1963; Beck, 1945, 1968, 1978; Bohm, 1958; Korchin, 1960; Mayman, 1970; Meyer & Caruth, 1970; Piotrowski, 1957; Schachtel, 1966).

SCHIZOPHRENIA

The schism in schizophrenia refers to the dissociation between thought and feeling—between cognitive processes and affect or emotional processes. A schizophrenic may have profoundly depressing kinds of thoughts without feeling depressed, or may become excited without apparent reason. Instances of the former type are more common and have given rise to the description of flattened affect in schizophrenia.

Schizophrenics are characterized by poor reality ties as well as the general symptoms of psychosis: hallucinations, delusions, disorientation, and bizarre behavior (see previous section). Numerous prodromal signs may herald an impending schizophrenic break with reality. Notable among these are impaired vocational performance, peculiar behavior such as collecting garbage, ideas of reference or clairvoyance, marked rambling or marginally coherent speech, and talking to oneself (American Psychiatric Association, 1980; Ullmann & Krasner, 1975; Weiner, 1966).

Behavioral Manifestations

Behavioral manifestations of schizophrenia include:

1. Withdrawn, socially distant behavior; close, warm, empathic relations are shunned for a more socially isolated and indifferent style of life.
2. Immature, regressive behavior.
3. Emotional blunting; even in the face of affect-arousing stimulation behavior is inappropriately unemotional.
4. Incoherent speech which may include neologisms, loose and/or clang associations, illogical syntax, and poverty of content.
5. Impaired personal hygiene.

Various other behavioral manifestations have been associated with specific forms or types of schizophrenia. Here we are content with general behavioral symptomatology which may be observed in any or all forms of the disorder. For descriptions of behavior associated with specific types of schizophrenia, the reader is referred to standard texts of abnormal psychology (Coleman, 1972; Martin, 1977; Ullmann & Krasner, 1975) and the DSM-III. Some behavioral symptoms of paranoid schizophrenia encompass symptoms of psychosis, of schizophrenia, and of paranoid disorders which are considered in the next section of this chapter. A comprehensive discussion of psychodiagnostics and schizophrenia can be found in Weiner's (1966) thorough book. Others have concluded, "If the clinician finds someone with hallucinations, delusions, and a thought disorder in the absence of gross organic findings, and without strong affective features, he [or she] is likely to diagnose such a person schizophrenic" (Bellak & Fielding, 1978, p. 757).

Test Indices

Wechsler Signs

1. **Verbal IQ significantly greater than Performance IQ** (Garfield, 1949; Gilbert, 1969; Goldfarb, 1961; Guertin et al., 1966; Gurvitz, 1951; Kahn & Giffen, 1960; Pope & Scott, 1967; Rabin, 1942; Sinnett & Mayman, 1960; Wechsler, 1958).
2. **Unusually low Information score** (Gilbert, 1969; Norman & Wilensky, 1961).
3. **Several misses on the early, easy Information items and more difficult items are passed** (Holt, 1968; Rapaport et al., 1945; Weiner, 1966).
4. **Particular difficulty with Information items 4, 5, 6, 9, 11, 13, 19, and 22** (Norman & Wilensky, 1961).
5. **Unusually high Information scores, especially with paranoid and preschizophrenic types** (Alexander, Crutchlow, & Hoffman, 1947; Bradway &

Benson, 1955; Gilbert, 1969; Holt, 1968; Magaret, 1942; Rabin, 1941, 1942; Wechsler, 1958; Zimmerman & Woo-Sam, 1973).

6. **Unusually low Comprehension scores, though paranoid types may not manifest this** (Alexander et al., 1947; DeWolfe, 1971; DeWolfe, Barrell, Becker, & Spaner, 1971; Gilbert, 1969; Gurvitz, 1951; Holt, 1968; Olch, 1948; Rapaport et al., 1945; Schafer, 1948; Weiner, 1966), **especially if the Envelope, Movies, and Forest items are failed** (Weiner, 1966).
7. **Low Comprehension score which is lower than the Digit Span score may differentiate schizophrenics from organics** (DeWolfe, 1971; DeWolfe et al., 1971).
8. **Comprehension scores significantly below Information scores** (Holt, 1968).
9. **Unusually high Digit Span scores, particularly if this score is higher than the Vocabulary score** (Allison et al., 1968; DeWolfe, 1971; DeWolfe et al., 1971; Gilbert, 1969; Holt, 1968; Keiser, 1975; Schafer, 1948; Watson, 1965).
10. **Digit Span score significantly above the Arithmetic score** (Allison, 1978; Allison et al., 1968; Blatt & Allison, 1968; Gurvitz, 1951; Holt, 1968; Rapaport et al., 1945; Schafer, 1948; Zimmerman & Woo-Sam, 1973).
11. **Significantly higher Digits Backward score than Digits Forward score** (Gilbert, 1969; Holt, 1968).
12. **Very significantly higher Digits Forward score than Digits Backward score** (Holt, 1968; Weiner, 1966).
13. **Unusually low Arithmetic score, especially when combined with a low Comprehension or Picture Arrangement score** (Glasser & Zimmerman, 1967; Gurvitz, 1951; Holt, 1968; Kahn & Giffen, 1960; Magaret, 1942; Rapaport et al., 1945; Schafer, 1948; Wechsler & Jaros, 1965).
14. **Unusually low Vocabulary score, though this may not hold for paranoid types** (Gilbert, 1969; Holt, 1968; Rapaport et al., 1945; Schafer, 1948).
15. **Unusually high Vocabulary score** (Bradway & Benson, 1955; Gilbert, 1969; Holt, 1968; Magaret, 1942; Wechsler, 1958; Zimmerman & Woo-Sam, 1973).
16. **Unusually low Similarities score** (Allison et al., 1968; Bradway & Benson, 1955; Gilbert, 1969; Holt, 1968; Kahn & Giffen, 1960; Pope & Scott, 1967; Rapaport et al., 1945; Wechsler, 1958; Weiner, 1966; Zimmerman & Woo-Sam, 1973).
17. **Unusually high Similarities subtest score, particularly with a low Picture Completion score** (Davis et al., 1972; Rapaport et al., 1945; Sat-

tler, 1974; Wechsler, 1958; Wechsler & Jaros, 1965).

18. **Overgeneralized, excessively inclusive Similarities responses such as "they both exist" or "both have molecules"** (Jortner, 1970; Weiner, 1966; Zimmerman & Woo-Sam, 1973), **or saying "They are not alike"** (Spence, 1963).

19. **Unusually low Picture Completion score** (Holt, 1968; Olch, 1948; Rapaport et al., 1945; Sattler, 1974; Wechsler, 1958; Wechsler & Jaros, 1965; Weiner, 1966).

20. **Unusually low Picture Arrangement score** (Alexander et al., 1947; Garfield, 1949; Gurvitz, 1951; Holt, 1968; Magaret, 1942; Olch, 1948; Rabin, 1942; Rapaport et al., 1945; Zimmerman & Woo-Sam, 1973).

21. **Unusually low Object Assembly score, particularly acute types** (Holt, 1968; Rabin, 1941; Weider, 1943).

22. **Unusually high Object Assembly score** (Bradway & Benson, 1955; Davis et al., 1972; Gurvitz, 1951; Holt, 1968; Rapaport et al., 1945; Sattler, 1974; Wechsler & Jaros, 1965; Zimmerman & Woo-Sam, 1973).

23. **Unusually high Block Design score** (Alexander et al., 1947; Allison et al., 1968; Bradway & Benson, 1955; Davis et al., 1972), **especially if Block Design is significantly greater than Picture Completion or Picture Arrangement** (Weiner, 1966).

24. **Unusually low Digit Symbol or Coding score** (Garfield, 1949; Heaton, Vogt, Hoehn, Lewis, Crowley, & Stallings, 1979; Holland et al., 1979; Holt, 1968; Magaret, 1942; Olch, 1948; Rabin, 1942; Rapaport et al., 1945; Wechsler & Jaros, 1965; Weiner, 1966; Zimmerman & Woo-Sam, 1973).

Rorschach Signs
Determinant Indices

1. **Very poor quality F responses** (Allen, 1954; Beck, 1944, 1945, 1951, 1968, 1978; Berkowitz & Levine, 1953; Bohm, 1958; DeVos, 1952; Dudek, 1969; Exner, 1974, 1978; Gottlieb & Parsons, 1960; Hertz & Paolino, 1960; Holt, 1968; Kahn & Giffen, 1960; Kalinowsky & Hoch, 1961; Kataguchi, 1959; Korchin, 1960; Molish, 1967; Neiger et al., 1962; Phillips & Smith, 1953; Piotrowski, 1957; Piotrowski & Berg, 1955; Piotrowski & Bricklin, 1961; Piotrowski & Lewis, 1950; Quinlan, Harrow, Tucker, & Carlson, 1972; Rapaport et al., 1946; Schaeffer, 1977; Schafer, 1948, 1954, 1960; Shapiro, 1977; Weiner, 1961b, 1966, 1977; Wolman, 1972).

2. **F% less than 20** (Beck, 1945; Piotrowski, 1957; Rapaport et al., 1946; Talkington & Reed, 1969; Vinson, 1960).

3. **M- responses present** (Beck, 1945; Exner, 1978; Hertz & Paolino, 1960; Molish, 1967; Mundy, 1972; Phillips & Smith, 1953; Schafer, 1960; Weiner, 1961b).

4. **Subnormal number of M** (Brar, 1970; Halpern, 1960; Kahn & Giffen, 1960; Piotrowski, 1960; Shapiro, 1977; Weiner, 1961b, 1966).

5. **FM- responses present, especially with paranoid schizophrenics** (Hertz & Paolino, 1960).

6. **Poor quality inanimate movement responses, especially with paranoid schizophrenics** (Hertz & Paolino, 1960).

7. **Subnormal number of FC** (Beck, 1945; Hughes, 1950; Molish, 1967; Rickers-Ovsiankina, 1954; Thiesen, 1952; Weiner, 1966).

8. **CF- responses present, especially in paranoid types** (Halpern, 1953; Hertz & Paolino, 1960; Mundy, 1972; Piotrowski, 1957; Shapiro, 1960).

9. **Pure C responses present** (Alcock, 1963; Allen, 1954; Beck, 1945; Exner, 1978; Kahn & Giffen, 1960; Molish, 1967; Mundy, 1972; Neuringer, 1962; Orme, 1966; Phillips & Smith, 1953; Powers & Hamlin, 1955; Rapaport et al., 1945; Rorschach, 1921/1951; Schachtel, 1966; Schafer, 1948; Shapiro, 1960, 1977; Vinson, 1960; Watkins & Stauffacher, 1952; Weiner, 1961b, 1964, 1966).

10. **Color naming responses present** (Alcock, 1963; Allen, 1954; Allison et al., 1968; Baker, 1956; Beck, 1945, 1978; Bohm, 1958; Brar, 1970; Halpern, 1953; Hughes, 1950; Kahn & Giffen, 1960; Neiger et al., 1962; Piotrowski, 1937b, 1957; Schachtel, 1966; Shapiro, 1977; Vinson, 1960; Weiner, 1966).

11. **FM greater than 2M or CF greater than FC** (Vinson, 1960).

12. **Sum C between 1 and 3.5** (Lambley, 1973; Weiner, 1961b, 1964, 1966).

13. **Sum C equal to zero** (Piotrowski & Berg, 1955; Piotrowski & Lewis, 1950; Shapiro, 1977).

14. **FC + CF + C approximately zero** (Bochner & Halpern, 1945; Bohm, 1958; Hertz, 1948, 1949; Piotrowski & Levine, 1959; Rapaport et al., 1946; Rorschach, 1921/1951; Schafer, 1960; Shapiro, 1960, 1977).

15. **CF or C responses without C'** (Weiner, 1961b, 1964, 1966).

16. **Sum C greater than 2M, particularly when M:Sum C is beyond 1:3 and M is 0 or 1** (Piotrowski & Bricklin, 1961; Rapaport et al., 1946; Schafer, 1948, 1954; Vinson, 1960).

17. *M + FC* equals zero (Thiesen, 1952).

18. **Subnormal number of texture-shading responses** (Kahn & Giffen, 1960; Piotrowski & Berg, 1955).

19. **Achromatic responses are greater than twice the number of chromatic responses** (Piotrowski & Levine, 1959; Piotrowski & Lewis, 1950).

20. **Sum *c* minus Sum *C* greater than three** (Piotrowski & Berg, 1955; Piotrowski & Lewis, 1950).

21. **Position responses present** (Alcock, 1963; Allison et al., 1968; Beck, 1944, 1945, 1978; Beck et al., 1961; Bohm, 1958; Dudek, 1969; Kelley & Klopfer, 1939; Piotrowski, 1957; Rorschach, 1921/ 1951; Watkins & Stauffacher, 1952; Weiner, 1966; Weiner & Exner, 1978).

22. **Number responses present; the number entirely justifies the response (e.g., "This is Mutt and Jeff, there were two of them and there are two of these")** (Piotrowski, 1957; Weiner, 1966).

23. **Unusually large number of reflection responses** (Exner, 1974, 1978).

24. **Unusually large number of pair (2) responses** (Exner, 1974, 1978).

25. **A color response to an achromatic area** (Beck, 1978).

Location Indices

1. **Subnormal number of *W*** (Goldfried et al., 1971; Piotrowski & Berg, 1955; Piotrowski & Levine, 1959; Siegel, 1953).

2. ***W-* or vague *W* responses are numerous** (Bohm, 1958; Friedman, 1952, 1953; Goldfried et al., 1971; Holt, 1968; Kataguchi, 1959; Kelley & Klopfer, 1939; Mundy, 1972; Piotrowski, 1957; Rapaport et al., 1946; Siegel, 1953; Weiner, 1966).

3. ***DW* responses present** (Alcock, 1963; Beck, 1945, 1978; Bochner & Halpern, 1945; Dudek, 1969; Exner, 1974; Friedman, 1953; Goldfried et al., 1971; Holt, 1968; Klopfer et al., 1954; Phillips & Smith, 1953; Piotrowski, 1957; Powers & Hamlin, 1955; Rapaport et al., 1946; Rorschach, 1921/ 1951; Schafer, 1948; Thiesen, 1952; Vinson, 1960; Watkins & Stauffacher, 1952).

4. ***D-* responses present** (Bohm, 1958; Friedman, 1953; Goldfried et al., 1971; Hertz & Paolino, 1960; Klopfer et al., 1954).

5. **Greater than normal number of *D*** (Halpern, 1960; Kalinowsky & Hoch, 1961; Weiner, 1966).

6. **Greater than normal number of small common detail responses with a subnormal number of *W*** (Piotrowski, 1957).

7. **Greater than normal number of *Dd* responses, especially when they are of poor form** (Bohm, 1958; Exner, 1974; Hertz & Paolino, 1960; Klopfer & Davidson, 1962; Piotrowski, 1957; Siegel, 1953; Vinson, 1960; Weiner, 1966).

8. **Greater than normal number of *dr* responses, especially with poor form level** (Allen, 1954, 1958; Hertz & Paolino, 1960; Holt, 1968; Klopfer et al., 1956; Knopf, 1956, 1965; Rapaport et al., 1946; Schafer, 1948, 1954; Siegel, 1953).

9. **Greater than normal number of *de* responses** (Phillips & Smith, 1953).

10. **Emphasis on *di* responses** (Klopfer & Davidson, 1962; Phillips & Smith, 1953).

11. **Greater than normal number of *S* responses** (Beck, 1945, 1960; Fonda, 1960; Hertz, 1948; Holt, 1968; Rapaport et al., 1946; Schafer, 1954).

Content Indices

1. **Few or no *A* responses, particularly with few or no large animals given** (Beck, 1945, 1952; Goldfried et al., 1971; Phillips & Smith, 1953; Rapaport et al., 1946; Thiesen, 1952).

2. **Greater than normal number of *A* content given, particularly if in excess of 50%** (Beck, 1945; Rapaport et al., 1946; Schafer, 1948; Vinson, 1960; Weiner, 1966).

3. **Greater than normal number of *Ad* responses, primarily seen in paranoid schizophrenics** (Allen, 1954).

4. **Weird, bizarre, deformed, or moribund animals** (Brar, 1970; DeVos, 1952; Mundy, 1972).

5. ***A* content with grasping claws, primarily seen in paranoid schizophrenia** (DeCourcy, 1971).

6. **Subnormal number, especially a void, of *H* responses** (Allison et al., 1968; Exner, 1978; Piotrowski & Bricklin, 1961; Weiner, 1966).

7. **(*H*) content in significant number** (Brar, 1970; DeCourcy, 1971; Exner, 1978; Lindner, 1947; Ritzler et al., 1980; Vinson, 1960; Weiner, 1966).

8. ***Hd* content of a front view face, primarily seen in paranoid types** (Bochner & Halpern, 1945; DuBrin, 1962; Phillips & Smith, 1953; Piotrowski, 1957).

9. ***Hd* content of biting teeth, primarily seen in paranoid types** (DeCourcy, 1971).

10. ***Hdx* and *Adx* content in significant number** (Phillips & Smith, 1953; Siegel, 1953).

11. ***AH* responses present** (Brar, 1970).

12. **Siamese twins content present** (Halpern, 1953).

13. ***H* content with *Dd* locations used** (Beck, 1945, 1960).

14. ***H + Hd* equal to zero** (Piotrowski, 1969).

15. *H + A* less than twice the (*Hd + Ad*) content (Rorschach, 1921/1951; Vinson, 1960).

16. *Hd* content of eyes, especially if peering or piercing, primarily in paranoid types (Alcock, 1963; Allen, 1954; Beck, 1960; Bochner & Halpern, 1945; Bradway & Heisler, 1953; DeCourcy, 1971; DuBrin, 1962; Due & Wright, 1945; Fonda, 1960; Kahn & Giffen, 1960; Klopfer et al., 1954; Lindner, 1946, 1947; Miale, 1947; Phillips & Smith, 1953; Piotrowski, 1957; Pope & Scott, 1967; Weiner, 1966).

17. Anatomy content to eight or more cards (Aronow & Reznikoff, 1976; Brar, 1970; DeVos, 1952; Exner, 1974; Goldfried et al., 1971; Knopf, 1956, 1965; Thiesen, 1952; Shereshevski-Shere, Lasser, & Gottesfeld, 1953; Weiner, 1966).

18. Visceral or soft anatomy content used (Beck, 1945; DeVos, 1952; Levitt & Truumaa, 1972; Phillips & Smith, 1953).

19. Crude anatomy responses such as "your guts" or "your insides" given (Beck, 1945; DeVos, 1952; Kalinowski & Hoch, 1961; Phillips & Smith, 1953).

20. Sex content in significant number (Beck, 1945; Carlson et al., 1973; DeVos, 1952; Due & Wright, 1945; Goldfried et al., 1971; Knopf, 1956, 1965; Molish, 1967; Orme, 1962; Phillips & Smith, 1953; Piotrowski, 1957; Potkay, 1971; Rapaport et al., 1946; Schafer, 1948; Thiesen, 1952; Vinson, 1960; Weiner, 1966).

21. Abstract content used in significant number (Bohm, 1958; Brar, 1970; Jortner, 1966; Kalinowsky & Hoch, 1961; Phillips & Smith, 1953; Quirk et al., 1962; Weiner, 1966).

22. Alphabet, numbers, punctuation, and geometric responses used (Bohm, 1958; Brar, 1970; Jortner, 1966; Klopfer & Davidson, 1962; Orme, 1963; Phillips & Smith, 1953; Piotrowski, 1957; Schafer, 1948, 1954; Weiner, 1966).

23. Blood content used in significant number (Brar, 1970; Rapaport et al., 1946; Schafer, 1948; Vinson, 1960).

24. Fire content used in significant number (Brar, 1970).

25. Food content used in significant number (Phillips & Smith, 1953; Schafer, 1948).

26. Teeth and gums content used in significant number (Phillips & Smith, 1953).

27. Mask content used, primarily in paranoid types (Beck, 1960; DuBrin, 1962; Vinson, 1960; Weiner, 1966).

28. Mutilated or other primitive, aggressive content given in significant number (Brar, 1970; Harrow et al., 1976).

29. Religion and supernatural content used in significant number (Jortner, 1966; Phillips & Smith, 1953; Weiner, 1966).

30. Urine stain response to yellow on Card X (Holt, 1968).

31. Water landscape content used in significant number (Brar, 1970).

32. Few content categories used (Allison et al., 1968; Evans & Marmorston, 1963; Olch, 1971; Piotrowski & Bricklin, 1961; Sherman, 1955).

33. Only one content category used (Allison et al., 1968; Beck, 1945; Brar, 1970).

34. Unusually high Anatomy + Sex content (DeVos, 1952; Taulbee & Sisson, 1954; Thiesen, 1952; Weiner, 1966).

Other Rorschach Indices

1. Subnormal number of *P* (Alcock, 1963; Allen, 1954; Beck, 1945, 1952, 1978; Berkowitz & Levine, 1953; Bloom, 1962; Bochner & Halpern, 1945; Bohm, 1958; Exner, 1974; Goldfried et al., 1971; Kataguchi, 1959; Knopf, 1956, 1965; Pierce et al., 1973; Schafer, 1948, 1960; Thiesen, 1952; Vinson, 1960; Weiner, 1966).

2. *O-* responses present (Alcock, 1963; Allen, 1954, 1958; Bochner & Halpern, 1945; Bohm, 1958; Hertz & Paolino, 1960; Kalinowski & Hoch, 1961; Klopfer et al., 1954; Miale, 1947; Pierce et al., 1973; Quirk et al., 1962; Rapaport et al., 1946; Rorschach, 1921/1951).

3. *O +* and *O-* responses in the same protocol (Kelley & Klopfer, 1939).

4. Subnormal number of *O* (Pierce et al., 1973).

5. Subnormal number of responses (Kahn & Giffen, 1960; Rickers-Ovsiankina, 1954; Schafer, 1960; Sherman, 1955), primarily in paranoid and simple types (Holt, 1968; Kahn & Giffen, 1960; Moylan, Shaw, & Appleman, 1960; Piotrowski, 1957; Weiner, 1966).

6. Greater than normal number of responses (Beck, 1951; Holt, 1968; Sherman, 1955).

7. Confabulations, abnormal content combinations or content that changes during the Performance (Brar, 1970; Dudek, 1969; Friedman, 1952, 1953; Goldfried et al., 1971; Jortner, 1966; Kahn & Giffen, 1960; Klopfer et al., 1954; Phillips & Smith, 1953; Pope & Scott, 1967; Rapaport et al., 1946; Schafer, 1948; Shapiro, 1977; Watkins & Stauffacher, 1952; Weiner, 1966; Weiner & Exner, 1978).

8. Confused sequence, less than three cards treated systematically (Allen, 1954).

9. **Edging observed** (Allen, 1954; Baker, 1956; Beck, 1945; Klopfer et al., 1954; Phillips & Smith, 1953).

10. **Fabulized combinations, content that is part one thing, part another** (Carlson et al., 1973; Exner, 1978; Friedman, 1952, 1953; Goldfried et al., 1971; Jortner, 1966; Quinlan & Harrow, 1974; Quinlan et al., 1972; Schaeffer, 1977; Shapiro, 1977; Weiner, 1966).

11. **Impotence expressions** (Vinson, 1960).

12. **Looking at the back of the card** (Klopfer et al., 1954; Phillips & Smith, 1953; Rapaport et al., 1946).

13. **Perplexity expressed** (Piotrowski, 1969; Vinson, 1960).

14. **Perseverations or repetitions** (Beck, 1945; Bohm, 1958; Dudek, 1969; Friedman, 1952, 1953; Hertz & Paolino, 1960; Kahn & Giffen, 1960; Klopfer et al., 1954; Piotrowski, 1969; Piotrowski & Bricklin, 1961; Schafer, 1948; Shapiro, 1977; Vinson, 1960; Weiner, 1966).

15. **Content has an unpleasant, dysphoric tone** (Brar, 1970).

16. **Shock to Card IV** (Berkowitz & Levine, 1953; Goldfried et al., 1971; Piotrowski, 1957; Piotrowski & Berg, 1955; Piotrowski & Lewis, 1950).

17. **Blocking or shock to Card V** (Bohm, 1958; Brown, 1953; Klopfer et al., 1954; McCully, 1971; Piotrowski, 1957).

18. **Rejection or failure of Card V** (Bochner & Halpern, 1945; Goldfried et al., 1971; Piotrowski & Berg, 1955; Piotrowski & Lewis, 1950; Weiner, 1966).

19. **Blocking or shock to Card VI** (Goldfried et al., 1971; Klopfer et al., 1954; Phillips & Smith, 1953; Piotrowski, 1957).

20. **Contaminations, where two associations are fused or connected, often with different determinants, in the same blot area** (Aronow & Reznikoff, 1976; Beck, 1978; Beck et al., 1961; Dudek, 1969; Exner, 1978; Klopfer et al., 1954, 1956; Powers & Hamlin, 1955; Quinlan & Harrow, 1974; Schaeffer, 1977; Shapiro, 1977; Weiner, 1966; Weiner & Exner, 1978).

21. **More responses to Card IX than to Card VIII** (Orme, 1964; Weiner, 1962, 1966).

22. **More responses to Card V than to Cards IV or VI** (Weiner, 1962, 1966).

23. **More responses to Card IX than to Card X** (Weiner, 1962, 1966).

24. **No human *P* response to Plate III or animal *P* to VIII** (Molish, 1951; Weiner, 1966).

Projective Drawing Signs
Graphological and General Indices

1. **Very light pressure used** (Hammer, 1958; Machover, 1949; Precker, 1950; Urban, 1963).

2. **Very tiny drawings made** (Buck, 1948; Hammer, 1969a; Kahn & Giffen, 1960; Machover, 1949; Urban, 1963).

3. **Short, discontinuous strokes used** (Small, 1973).

4. **Gross distortions in drawings** (Burton & Sjoberg, 1964; Hozier, 1959; Jacks, 1969; Kahn & Giffen, 1960; McElhaney, 1969).

5. **Extreme bilateral symmetry with very mechanical, formalistic, or bizarre effects produced, especially noted in paranoid types** (Machover, 1949; Urban, 1963).

6. **Omissions of essential details of normals' drawings** (see Chapter 2 on Normality) (Buck, 1948; Deabler, 1969; Kahn & Giffen, 1960; Ries et al., 1966; Swensen, 1968).

Draw-A-Person/Human Figure Drawing Indices

1. **Unusually large head drawn, especially by males** (Baldwin, 1964; Burton & Sjoberg, 1964).

2. **Head only drawn for the drawing of a person** (Baldwin, 1964; Schildkrout et al., 1972).

3. **Eyes omitted** (Deabler, 1969; Hammer, 1969a).

4. **Two eyes depicted in a profile drawing** (Gilbert, 1969).

5. **Hair omitted from the human figure drawing** (Hammer, 1969a; Holzberg & Wexler, 1950; Hozier, 1959).

6. **Teeth showing in drawing** (Buck, 1964, 1966; Hammer, 1958; Jolles, 1971; Koppitz, 1968; Levy, 1950, 1958; Machover, 1949; McElhaney, 1969; Schildkrout et al., 1972; Urban, 1963).

7. **Nonhuman or animal or other bizarre facial features on the drawing of a person** (McElhaney, 1969).

8. **Exceptionally long, thin necks** (Buck, 1964, 1966, 1969; Gurvitz, 1951; Hammer, 1954c; Jolles, 1971; Levy, 1950, 1958; Machover, 1949; Urban, 1963).

9. **A dehumanized human figure; torso as boxy, automaton or robot-like, square or other geometric shape** (Chase, 1941; Hammer, 1978; McElhaney, 1969; Ries et al., 1966).

10. **Shoulders absent from drawn person** (Burton & Sjoberg, 1964; Holzberg & Wexler, 1950).

11. **Arms omitted from drawn person** (Buck, 1966; DeLeo, 1973; Gilbert, 1969; Gurvitz, 1951; Hammer, 1954c; Holzberg & Wexler, 1950; Jolles, 1969, 1971; Kahn & Giffen, 1960; Kokonis,

1972; Koppitz, 1968; Levy, 1958; Machover, 1949; Urban, 1963).

12. **Wing-like arms** (Buck, 1966; Hammer, 1954c, 1978; Jolles, 1971; Machover, 1958; Urban, 1963).

13. **Joints emphasized, especially by paranoid types** (Hammer, 1968; Kahn & Giffen, 1960; Machover, 1949, 1951, 1955; Roback, 1968; Urban, 1963; Wildman, 1963).

14. **Omission of hands** (Buck, 1948, 1964, 1966; DiLeo, 1973; Gilbert, 1969; Hammer, 1958; Mundy, 1972; Mursell, 1969; Schildkrout et al., 1972; Urban, 1963; Weiner, 1966).

15. **Breasts omitted** (Burton & Sjoberg, 1964).

16. **Unusually large breasts drawn on females by a male** (Ries et al., 1966).

17. **Omission of feet** (Buck, 1948, 1950, 1966; Hammer, 1954c; Jolles, 1971; Kokonis, 1972; Schildkrout et al., 1972; Urban, 1963).

18. **Stiff posture drawn, especially by paranoid types** (Kahn & Giffen, 1960).

19. **Genitalia drawn** (Deabler, 1969; Gilbert, 1969; Kahn & Giffen, 1960; Machover, 1951; Urban, 1963; Weiner, 1966).

20. **Underclothed or nude figure drawn** (Hammer, 1968; Holzberg & Wexler, 1950; Machover, 1949; Urban, 1963; Weiner, 1966).

21. **Transparent clothing drawn** (Holzberg & Wexler, 1950; Hozier, 1959; Machover, 1949; McElhaney, 1969; Reynolds, 1978; Weiner, 1966).

22. **Buttons emphasized** (Ries et al., 1966).

23. **A row of irrelevant buttons drawn down the midline of human figure drawing** (Hammer, 1954c; Machover, 1949, 1955; Schildkrout et al., 1972; Urban, 1963).

24. **Clear indications of internal organs in drawing of a person** (Buck, 1966; Kahn & Giffen, 1960; Levy, 1950, 1958; Machover, 1949, 1951; McElhaney, 1969; Urban, 1963; Weiner, 1966).

25. **Refusal to draw the human figure below the waist, or at most only a few sketchy lines are used** (Buck, 1966; Jolles, 1971; Kokonis, 1972; Machover, 1949; Urban, 1963).

26. **Back of person drawn** (Gilbert, 1969; McElhaney, 1969).

27. **Confusion of profile and full face** (Gilbert, 1969; Kahn & Giffen, 1960; Machover, 1949; Urban, 1963).

28. **Figure drawn to suggest whirling movement** (Schildkrout et al., 1972).

29. **A fragmented human figure is drawn** (Weiner, 1961b).

H-T-P House and Tree Drawing Indices

1. **House drawn with a double perspective with both end walls exaggerated** (Buck, 1948; Deabler, 1969; Hammer, 1954c; Jolles, 1971).

2. **House drawn only as a roof (not as an A-frame dwelling)** (Buck, 1964; Deabler, 1969; Hammer, 1954c, 1958).

3. **House drawn very small** (Buck, 1948).

4. **Tree drawn as two one-dimensional trees side by side, each with an independent branch structure** (Buck, 1948; Deabler, 1969; Hammer, 1954c, 1958, 1978; Jacks, 1969; Jolles, 1971; Koch, 1952; Landisberg, 1958; Levine & Sapolsky, 1969).

5. **Tree drawn dead** (Hammer, 1958).

6. **An anthropomorphic house is drawn** (Hammer, 1978).

Bender-Gestalt Signs
Unusual Reproduction Modes and Arrangements

1. **Very tiny reproductions** (Allen, 1958; Bender, 1938; Gilbert, 1969; Guertin, 1955).

2. **Very large reproductions** (Goldberg, 1956-57; Guertin, 1954a; Kahn & Giffen, 1960; Woltmann, 1950).

3. **Concreteness, reproducing the figures with specific interpretive meaning** (Halpern, 1951; Kahn & Giffen, 1960).

4. **Displacement; the parts of a gestalt are related in a bizarre way** (Halpern, 1951).

5. **Destruction of the gestalt is accomplished by spontaneous elaborations, etc.** (Bender, 1938; Hutt, 1953, 1968, 1977; Hutt & Gibby, 1970; Woltmann, 1950).

6. **Fragmentation** (Allen, 1958; Bender, 1938; Clawson, 1962; Gilbert, 1969; Guertin, 1954a; Halpern, 1951; Hutt, 1953, 1968, 1977; Hutt & Briskin, 1960; Hutt & Gibby, 1970; Woltmann, 1950).

7. **Lines changed to dots** (Allen, 1958).

8. **Overlapping and crossing difficulty** (Bender, 1938; Gilbert, 1969; Goldberg, 1956-57; Halpern, 1951; Hutt & Gibby, 1970; Koppitz, 1958).

9. **Perseverations** (Bender, 1938; Gilbert, 1969; Goldberg, 1956-57; Hutt, 1953, 1977; Hutt & Gibby, 1970; Piotrowski, 1957).

10. **Regression, including simplification, primitivation, and condensation** (Bender, 1938; Gilbert, 1969; Goldberg, 1956-57; Guertin, 1952; Halpern, 1951; Hutt, 1953, 1968, 1977; Hutt & Gibby, 1970; Woltmann, 1950).

11. **Reversals and rotations** (Bender, 1938; Hutt, 1977)

12. **Turning cards or paper** (Hutt, 1968).

13. **A confused or chaotic arrangement** (Bender, 1938; Goldberg, 1956-57; Guertin, 1954c; Halpern, 1951; Hutt, 1953, 1968, 1977; Hutt & Briskin, 1960).

14. **Crowded, compressed, cohesive arrangements** (Bender, 1938; Gilbert, 1969; Goldberg, 1956-57; Guertin, 1955; Halpern, 1951; Hutt, 1968, 1977).

15. **Closure difficulty** (Hutt, 1977).

16. **The total figure is redrawn** (Hutt, 1977).

Unusual Treatment of Specific Figures

1. **Poor circle form in Figure A** (Goldberg, 1956-57).

2. **Abnormal placement of Figure A** (Hutt, 1968, 1977).

3. **Treating the two parts of Figure A as if they were independent units rather than parts of one gestalt** (Halpern, 1951).

4. **Rotation and gross disorganization of Figure A** (Guertin, 1952).

5. **General difficulty with Figure 1** (Hutt & Briskin, 1960).

6. **Perseveration on Figures 1 and 2** (Bender, 1938; Goldberg, 1956-57; Halpern, 1951; Koppitz, 1962; Weissman & Roth, 1965).

7. **Horizontal direction lost with Figure 2 acquiring a curve above or below the initial base** (Halpern, 1951; Hutt & Briskin, 1960).

8. **Perseveration and number distortion on Figure 2** (Bender, 1938; Lerner, 1972).

9. **On Figure 3 the center dots are not level with a loss of angles** (Guertin, 1954c).

10. **A flock of birds drawn as a concrete reproduction of Figure 3** (Halpern, 1951).

11. **Nonclosure of Figure 4 related to difficulty with the curvilinear element** (Guertin, 1952; Lerner, 1972).

12. **On Figure 6 the crossing point located incorrectly** (Guertin, 1954c).

13. **On Figure 6 excessive waves reproduced** (Guertin, 1952).

14. **Reproducing Figure 7 as two independent units, which may also be noted in Figure A** (Halpern, 1951).

15. **Poor, inappropriate angulation on Figure 7** (Guertin, 1954c).

Contraindications

1. **Unusually high number of *FC* responses on the Rorschach** (Beck, 1945).

2. **Frequent erasures on projective drawings** (Ogdon, 1975).

PARANOID SUSPICIOUSNESS AND PARANOIA

Various paranoid disorders are marked essentially by expressions of false ideas that are maintained. Speech reveals the suspiciousness and delusional processes. Since this is essentially a disorder of cognition, it is quite difficult to enumerate behavioral manifestations which are clearly and univocally pertinent. Overt manifestations, when present, tend to be secondary symptoms at best. The primary symptom of all paranoid individuals is a false conviction or belief which is unshakable and impervious to logic. Paranoid symptoms appear to grow out of a psychological orientation of suspicion, wariness of the motives of others, and hypersensitivity. The defense of projection may contribute by fostering a hostile attitude toward others. This hostility directly results from perceiving one's own ego-alien tendencies in others. When delusional ideation occurs with symptoms of schizophrenia, there may be paranoid schizophrenia. When false ideas occur without symptoms of psychosis, there may be a paranoid personality or other paranoid condition.

Typically the delusion of reference occurs earliest. An individual mistakenly thinks some environmental action has personal meaning. Normal people make this kind of mistake, but normals will correct the mistaken idea when evidence appears or logic suggests they were in error. Paranoids fail to make the correction. Subsequently, they will develop delusions of persecution or of being controlled by others as a function of projecting their own ego-alien desire to control or take advantage of others. Finally, delusions of self-aggrandizement will become necessary to explain why they have been singled out for the unusual attention and persecution they have experienced.

Behavioral Manifestations

Behavioral manifestations of paranoid disorders include verbal references to:

1. People watching them.

2. People or forces trying to influence or control their thoughts or behavior.

3. People taking advantage of them or trying to persecute them in other ways.

4. Inflated ideas of self-importance and grandiose plans, etc.

It should be noted that legal proceedings and homosexual proclivities are frequent epiphenomena of paranoia.

Test Indices

Wechsler Signs

1. **Unusually high Information scores** (Alexander et al., 1947; Bradway & Benson, 1955; Gilbert, 1969; Holt, 1968; Magaret, 1942; Rabin, 1941, 1942; Wechsler, 1958).
2. **Unusually high Comprehension scores** (Gilbert, 1969; Holt, 1968; Rabin, 1941, 1942; Wittenborn & Holzberg, 1951).
3. **Unusually high Similarities scores accompanied by high Arithmetic and high Picture Completion scores** (Allison, 1978; Allison et al., 1968; Gilbert, 1969; Holt, 1968; Rapaport et al., 1945; Schafer, 1948).
4. **Unusually high Arithmetic scores** (Gurvitz, 1951).
5. **Unusually high Picture Completion scores** (Allison, 1978; Allison et al., 1968; Gilbert, 1969; Holt, 1968; Zimmerman & Woo-Sam, 1973).
6. **Unusually high Picture Arrangement scores** (Allison, 1978; Allison et al., 1968; Gilbert, 1969).
7. **Unusually low Block Design scores** (Bradway & Benson, 1955).

Rorschach Signs

Determinant and Location Indices

1. **F% greater than 50** (Holt, 1968; Schafer, 1948).
2. **CF- responses present** (Halpern, 1953; Hertz & Paolino, 1960; Mundy, 1972; Piotrowski, 1957; Shapiro, 1960).
3. **M determinants with (H) content** (Phillips & Smith, 1953).
4. **M determinants with Hd content when the Hd are faces and eyes** (Phillips & Smith, 1953).
5. **Pure C responses present** (Hertz & Paolino, 1960; Rapaport et al., 1946; Shapiro, 1960).
6. **C symbolism responses present** (Miale, 1947).
7. **S responses emphasized, especially in coarctated records** (Beck, 1945, 1960; Fonda, 1960; Hertz, 1948; Holt, 1968; Rapaport et al., 1946; Schafer, 1954).
8. **Abnormally high number of de locations used** (Phillips & Smith, 1953).
9. **Sum of Dd + S responses abnormally high** (Alcock, 1963; Phillips & Smith, 1953).

Content and Other Rorschach Indices

1. **Eye content emphasized, especially if "peering" or "piercing"** (Alcock, 1963; Allen, 1954; Beck, 1945, 1960, 1978; Bochner & Halpern, 1945; Bradway & Heisler, 1953; DeCourcy, 1971; DuBrin, 1962; Endicott, Jortner, & Abramoff, 1969; Fonda, 1960; Kahn & Giffen, 1960; Klopfer et al., 1954; Klopfer & Davidson, 1962; Lindner, 1946, 1947; Miale, 1947; Phillips & Smith, 1953; Piotrowski, 1957; Pope & Scott, 1967; Weiner, 1966).
2. **Hd's as front views of faces noted** (Bochner & Halpern, 1945; DuBrin, 1962; Endicott et al., 1969; Phillips & Smith, 1953; Piotrowski, 1957), **or as fingers pointing** (Endicott et al., 1969).
3. **Ear content emphasized** (Miale, 1947).
4. **Biting teeth content present** (DeCourcy, 1971).
5. **Anus or buttocks content, especially if associated with peering eyes** (Aronson, 1952; Beck, 1945; Klopfer & Davidson, 1962; Miale, 1947; Pascal, Ruesch, Devine, & Suttell, 1950; Piotrowski, 1957).
6. **Mask content emphasized** (Beck, 1960; DuBrin, 1962; Endicott et al., 1969; Vinson, 1960).
7. **Religion content emphasized** (Aronson, 1952; Miale, 1947).
8. **Abnormally large number of A responses** (Schafer, 1948).
9. **Abnormally large number of Ad responses** (Allen, 1954).
10. **Abnormally long reaction and response times** (Allen, 1954; Piotrowski, 1957).
11. **Looking at the back of the card** (Allen, 1954; Klopfer et al., 1954; Phillips & Smith, 1953).
12. **Rejections or failures present** (Allison et al., 1968; Bochner & Halpern, 1945; Hertz, 1948; Holt, 1968; Schafer, 1954).
13. **Blocking or shock to Card I** (Klopfer et al., 1954; Piotrowski, 1957).
14. **Threatening content, especially such as H or A as a W to Plate IV** (Aronson, 1952; Endicott et al., 1969).
15. **Devil, demon, witch content or H content dressed in capes, cloaks, armor, and clown or other costumes** (Endicott et al., 1969).
16. **H content described as evil, sinister, crafty, dishonest, etc.** (Endicott et al., 1969).
17. **H content persecuting, torturing, or attempting to control another human** (Endicott et al., 1969).

Projective Drawing Signs

Graphological and General Indices

1. **Very large drawings** (Machover, 1949; McElhaney, 1969; Urban, 1963; Weiner, 1966).
2. **Very heavy pressure used** (Hammer, 1958; Reznikoff & Nicholas, 1958; Roback, 1968; Weiner, 1966).
3. **Very light pressure used** (Hammer, 1958; Machover, 1949; Precker, 1950; Urban, 1963).

Draw-A-Person/Human Figure Drawing Indices

1. **Abnormally large head** (Machover, 1949, 1951; Urban, 1963).
2. **Eyes drawn abnormally large or strongly reinforced** (Deabler, 1969; Gilbert, 1969; Griffith & Peyman, 1959; Hammer, 1954c, 1978; Jacks, 1969; Kahn & Giffen, 1960; Levy, 1950, 1958; Machover, 1949, 1951, 1958; McElhaney, 1969; Reznikoff & Nicholas, 1958; Schildkrout et al., 1972; Urban, 1963).
3. **Eyes drawn on the side of the head** (Schildkrout et al., 1972).
4. **Ears drawn abnormally large or strongly reinforced** (Griffith & Peyman, 1959; Hammer, 1978; Jacks, 1969; Levine & Sapolsky, 1969; Levy, 1950, 1958; Landisberg, 1969; Machover, 1949, 1951; McElhaney, 1969; Schildkrout et al., 1972; Urban, 1963).
5. **Ears drawn as questions marks** (McElhaney, 1969).
6. **Earrings emphasized** (McElhaney, 1969).
7. **Arms and legs drawn pressed to the body as if to ward off the environment** (Hammer, 1958; Machover, 1949).
8. **Arms drawn folded** (Buck, 1964, 1966; Hammer, 1954c; Jolles, 1971; Urban, 1963).
9. **Fingers drawn as talon-like spikes or dark straight lines** (Brown, 1958; Buck, 1964, 1966; Goldstein & Rawn, 1957; Hammer, 1954c, 1958, 1965; Jacks, 1969; Jolles, 1971; Machover, 1949; McElhaney, 1969; Schildkrout et al., 1972; Shneidman, 1958; Urban, 1963; Wolk, 1969).
10. **Figure drawn in absolute profile with only one arm and one leg visible** (Buck, 1964; Hammer, 1954c; McElhaney, 1969).
11. **Back of person drawn to viewer** (Hammer, 1954c; Jacks, 1969; McElhaney, 1969).
12. **Joints of body emphasized** (Hammer, 1968; Kahn & Giffen, 1960; Machover, 1949, 1951, 1955; Roback, 1968; Urban, 1963; Wildman, 1963).
13. **Hip emphasized** (Machover, 1951; Urban, 1963).
14. **Hands drawn inserted in pockets** (DiLeo, 1973; Jolles, 1971; Machover, 1949; McElhaney, 1969; Schildkrout et al., 1972; Urban, 1963).

H-T-P House and Tree Drawing Indices

1. **Only one side wall drawn for a house** (Buck, 1948, 1964, 1966; Hammer, 1958; Jolles, 1971).
2. **A blueprint or floor plan drawn for a house** (Hammer, 1954c; Jacks, 1969; Jolles, 1971).
3. **Eaves emphasized in House drawing** (Buck, 1966; Hammer, 1954c; Mursell, 1969).
4. **Rear of house drawn** (Jolles, 1971).
5. **Doors drawn with heavy hinges** (Buck, 1948; Hammer, 1958; Jolles, 1971).
6. **Rain spouts and gutters drawn on house** (Buck, 1964; Hammer, 1954c; Jolles, 1971).
7. **Tree drawing is a fruit tree** (Marzolf & Kirchner, 1972).
8. **Talon-like roots drawn** (Buck, 1964, 1966; Hammer, 1954c; Jolles, 1971).

Bender-Gestalt Signs

1. **Excessive workover of reproductions** (Pascal & Suttell, 1951; Woltmann, 1950).
2. **Numbering and boxing-off of reproductions** (Gilbert, 1969).
3. **Sketching** (Pascal & Suttell, 1951).
4. **Small reproductions made with excessive space between the figures, a scattered arrangement** (DeCato & Wicks, 1976; Hutt, 1953, 1978; Hutt & Briskin, 1960).
5. **Extremely compressed arrangement** (DeCato & Wicks, 1976; Guertin, 1955).
6. **Irregular arrangement** (Guertin, 1955).
7. **Numerous sheets of paper are required** (Brown, 1965; Clawson, 1962).
8. **General difficulty reproducing Figure 1** (Hutt & Briskin, 1960).
9. **The pairing of dots emphasized on Figure 1** (Lerner, 1972).
10. **Elaboration of curves on Figure 6 as a face or insertion of a dot for an eye** (Hutt, 1977; Hutt & Briskin, 1960).
11. **Edge placement** (Hutt, 1977).
12. **Overextension of secant on Figure 5** (Hutt, 1977).

MANIC-DEPRESSIVE DISORDERS

Among the functional psychoses, affective disorders are generally considered to manifest less severe personality disorganization and to have a better prognosis than schizophrenia. Manics and depressives may be expected to respond reasonably well to a variety of psychotherapeutic techniques and psycho-pharmacological agents. The primary dangers to prevent are violent destructiveness during maniacal episodes and suicide during depressive periods. Test indices of acting out tendencies, noted in Chapter 5, should prove helpful in this regard.

From our point of view there are four subgroups of manic-depressive conditions: manic, depressive, circular, and mixed types. Test indices enumerated below are in three groups: signs suggesting the presence of an affective disorder, signs of manic conditions, and signs of depressive conditions. Diagnoses of other classes of affective disorders may be achieved by using combinations of signs. For instance, indices of both mania and depression would suggest a circular or mixed type. Indices of neurosis along with depressive signs would suggest depressive neurosis, etc.

More thorough developmental descriptions of these disorders, relevant theoretical considerations, and differential responses to therapy are available elsewhere in the literature (American Psychiatric Association, 1980; Coleman, 1972; Martin, 1977; Ullmann & Krasner, 1975; Wolman, 1978).

Behavioral Manifestations

Behavioral manifestations of *mania*, approximately in order of increasing severity, include:
1. Loquacious, flighty, boisterous, and grandiose speech.
2. Inflated self-esteem and a tendency toward an elated grandiosity.
3. Excessive activity in inappropriate business ventures, sexual escapades, reckless driving, etc.
4. Confused, vulgar, obscene, and incoherent speech.
5. Disturbed sleep patterns.
6. High distractibility and extreme hyperactivity.
7. Unpredictable violent and destructive behavior.

Behavioral manifestations of *depression*, approximately in order of increasing severity, include:
1. Slowing of speech and other activity.
2. Negativism.
3. Frequent expression of guilt, sorrow, and dysphoric mood.
4. Complaints of easy fatigability.
5. Abulia, chronic indecisiveness.
6. Disturbances of eating, anorexia, or bulimia.
7. Disturbances of sleeping, insomnia, or hypersomnia.
8. Mutism.
9. Death wishes expressed or suicide contemplated seriously or attempted.

Test Indices of an Affective Disorder

Wechsler Signs
1. **Unusually low Digit Span score** (Alexander et al., 1947; Gilbert, 1969; Glasser & Zimmerman, 1967; Holt, 1968; Rabin, 1942; Schafer, 1948).

Rorschach Signs
1. **Subnormal number of *M*** (Alcock, 1963; Hertz, 1948, 1949; Piotrowski, 1957; Rapaport et al., 1946; Rorschach, 1921/1951; Schachtel, 1966; Schafer, 1948).

2. **Greater than normal number of *Ad* responses** (Allen, 1954; Bohm, 1958).

Projective Drawing Signs
1. **Human figure drawn with an abnormally large head** (McElhaney, 1969).
2. **Preoccupation with sexual detail** (Zimmerman & Garfinkle, 1942).

Bender-Gestalt Signs
1. **Rotations present** (Fuller & Chagnon, 1962; Guertin, 1952; Halpern, 1951; Hutt, 1953; Hutt & Gibby, 1970; Murray & Roberts, 1956).
2. **Spontaneous elaborations or embellishments present** (Bender, 1938; Gilbert, 1969; Hutt, 1953; Hutt & Briskin, 1960; Hutt & Gibby, 1970; Woltmann, 1950).
3. **Irregular arrangements** (Murray & Roberts, 1956).

Test Indices of a Manic Disorder

Wechsler Signs
1. **Unusually low Digit Symbol score** (Rabin, 1942).

Rorschach Signs
Determinant and Location Indices
1. **Subnormal quality *F* responses** (Beck, 1945; Korchin, 1960; Pope & Scott, 1967; Rapaport et al., 1946).
2. **$F\%$ less than 20** (Beck, 1945, 1951).
3. **CF- responses present** (Shapiro, 1960), **or *C/F*** (Shapiro, 1977).
4. **Sum *C* greater than 3** (Beck, 1945; Cerbus & Nichols, 1963; Shapiro, 1977).
5. **Sum *C* approximately equal to *M* and both are overemphasized** (Beck, 1960; Gurvitz, 1951; Rorschach, 1921/1951; Singer, 1960).
6. **An abnormally large number of *W* responses** (Beck, 1945; Bohm, 1958; Hertz, 1960; Piotrowski, 1957).
7. **A significant number of *di* responses present** (Allen, 1954).

Other Rorschach Indices
1. **Abstract content in significant number** (Brar, 1970).
2. **An abnormally large number of responses** (Alcock, 1963; Allen, 1954; Beck, 1945; Pope & Scott, 1967; Rorschach, 1921/1951).
3. **Abnormally short reaction times** (Allen, 1954; Bochner & Halpern, 1945; Kahn & Giffen, 1960).

4. **Responses with a pleasant or excited tone predominate** (Brar, 1970).

5. **Contaminations, abnormal thought combinations present** (Beck, 1945; Beck et al., 1961; Schafer, 1948).

6. **Confused (less than three systematic) sequences** (Allen, 1954).

Projective Drawing Signs

1. **Drawings are very large** (Hammer, 1969a; Kadis, 1950; Machover, 1949; McElhaney, 1969; Urban, 1963).

2. **Extreme excessive detailing of drawings** (Buck, 1966; McElhaney, 1969).

3. **Extreme asymmetry in human figure drawing** (Hammer, 1965, 1969b; Koppitz, 1966c; Machover, 1949; Mundy, 1972; Urban, 1963).

4. **Clear indications of internal organs in human figure drawing** (Buck, 1966; Kahn & Giffen, 1960; Levy, 1950, 1958; Machover, 1949, 1951; McElhaney, 1969; Urban, 1963).

5. **Tree drawing with excessive branches and leaves** (Levine & Sapolsky, 1969).

Bender-Gestalt Signs

1. **Abnormally large reproductions** (Gilbert, 1969).
2. **Closure difficulty** (Pascal & Suttell, 1951).
3. **Upward sloping of Bender figures** (Halpern, 1951; Weissman & Roth, 1965).
4. **Scattered, expansive arrangements** (Murray & Roberts, 1956).
5. **Confused or chaotic arrangements** (Murray & Roberts, 1956).
6. **On Figure 2, a loss of the horizontal direction so the figure curves above the original base** (Halpern, 1951; Hutt & Briskin, 1960).
7. **Spontaneous elaborations, embellishments, and doodling** (Bender, 1938; Hutt, 1953; Hutt & Briskin, 1960; Hutt & Gibby, 1970; Woltmann, 1950).
8. **Perseveration of curves on Figure 6** (DeCato & Wicks, 1976).

Test Indices of a Depressive Disorder

Wechsler Signs

1. **Unusually low Comprehension scores** (Alexander et al., 1947; Gilbert, 1969; Rapaport et al., 1945; Schafer, 1948; Weiner, 1966).

2. **A Comprehension score significantly below the Information score** (Holt, 1968).

3. **Unusually low Similarities score** (Alexander et al., 1947; Gilbert, 1969; Rapaport et al., 1945).

4. **Significantly more Digits Forward recited than Digits Backward** (Holt, 1968).

5. **Unusually low Digit Symbol score** (Allison, 1978; Allison et al., 1968; Blatt & Allison, 1968; Gilbert, 1969; Gurvitz, 1951; Henrichs & Amolsch, 1978; Holt, 1968; Pope & Scott, 1967; Rapaport et al., 1945; Schafer, 1948; Zimmerman & Woo-Sam, 1973).

6. **Unusually low Picture Arrangement score** (Alexander et al., 1947; Blatt & Quinlan, 1967; Holt, 1968; Rapaport et al., 1945; Zimmerman & Woo-Sam, 1973).

7. **Unusually low Object Assembly score** (Allison et al., 1968; Gurvitz, 1951; Henrichs & Amolsch, 1978; Holt, 1968; Rapaport et al., 1945).

8. **Unusually low Block Design score** (Henrichs & Amolsch, 1978; Holt, 1968; Rapaport et al., 1945; Schafer, 1948).

9. **VIQ significantly above the PIQ** (Alexander et al., 1947; Allison, 1978; Allison et al., 1968; Blatt & Allison, 1968; Guertin et al., 1966; Gurvitz, 1951; Henrichs & Amolsch, 1978; Holt, 1968; Schafer, 1948; Sinnett & Mayman, 1960; Zimmerman & Woo-Sam, 1973).

Rorschach Signs
Determinant Indices

1. **Subnormal number of *M* responses** (Alcock, 1963; Exner, 1974; Hertz, 1948, 1949; Piotrowski, 1957; Rapaport et al., 1946; Rorschach, 1921/1951; Schachtel, 1966; Schafer, 1948; Weiner, 1966).

2. **Flexor *M* responses emphasized** (Bochner & Halpern, 1945; Hertz, 1949; Pope & Scott, 1967; Taulbee, 1961).

3. ***M* determinants with *Hd* content** (Beck, 1945; Phillips & Smith, 1953).

4. ***F% greater than 50*** (Alcock, 1963; Allison et al., 1968; Bohm, 1958; Exner, 1974; Goldfried et al., 1971; Hertz, 1965; Levitt & Truumaa, 1972).

5. ***F* responses with better than average quality** (Allison et al., 1968; Beck, 1945, 1951; Holt, 1968; Korchin, 1960; Levi, 1951; Rorschach, 1921/1951).

6. **Greater than normal number of achromatic responses** (Alcock, 1963; Allen, 1954; Allison et al., 1968; Ames et al., 1959; Arnaud, 1959; Beck, 1945, 1951; Beck et al., 1961; Bochner & Halpern, 1945; Bohm, 1960; Brown, Chase, & Winson, 1961; Exner, 1978; Hafner & Rosen, 1964; Halpern, 1953; Kahn & Giffen, 1960; Klopfer et al., 1954; Miale, 1977; Molish, 1967; Rosenzweig & Kogan, 1949; Schafer, 1954; Wagner, 1971).

7. **Greater than normal number of Vista responses** (Exner, 1969a, 1974; Klopfer et al., 1954).

8. *KF + K* **in greater than normal number** (Alcock, 1963; Bochner & Halpern, 1945; Sarason, 1954).

9. *CF + C* **abnormally high and greater than** *FC* (Siegal et al., 1962).

10. *FC + CF + C* **approximately zero** (Bochner & Halpern, 1945; Bohm, 1958; Cerbus & Nichols, 1963; Exner, 1974; Hertz, 1948, 1949, 1965; Piotrowski & Levine, 1959; Rapaport et al., 1946; Rorschach, 1921/1951; Schafer, 1960; Shapiro, 1960; Weiner, 1961a).

11. **Sum** *C* **approximately equal to** *M* **and both are underemphasized** (Beck, 1960; Gurvitz, 1951; Palmer & Lustgarten, 1962; Rapaport et al., 1946; Rickers-Ovsiankina, 1960; Rorschach, 1921/1951; Schafer, 1948; Weiner, 1961a).

12. *F* **greater than 3** *(M + FM + FC + CF + C + Fc)* (Beck, 1960).

13. **Achromatic responses are greater than twice the number of chromatic** (Klopfer & Kelley, 1942; Sarason, 1954).

14. **Sum** *C* **is between 1 and 3.5** (Cerbus & Nichols, 1963; Cutter, Jorgenson, & Farberow, 1968; Daston & Sakheim, 1960; Goldfried et al., 1971; Rapaport et al., 1946; Weiner, 1961a).

15. **Greater than normal number of shading responses** (Elstein, 1965; Rickers-Ovsiankina, 1960).

16. *M* **responses with** *Hd* **content** (Beck, 1945; Phillips & Smith, 1953).

17. **Subnormal number of pair and reflection responses** (Exner, 1974, 1978; Exner & Wylie, 1977).

Location and Content Indices

1. **Subnormal number of** *W* **responses** (Beck, 1960; Bohm, 1958; Exner, 1974; Holt, 1968; Piotrowski, 1957; Rapaport et al., 1946; Rorschach, 1921/1951; Schafer, 1948).

2. **Abnormally large number of** *D* **responses** (Alcock, 1963; Beck, 1945; Weiner, 1961a).

3. **Presence of** *do* **responses** (Allen, 1954; Allison et al., 1968; Ames et al., 1952, 1974; Auerbach & Spielberger, 1972; Beck, 1945; Bochner & Halpern, 1945; Bohm, 1958; Eichler, 1951; Holt, 1968; Piotrowski, 1957; Rapaport et al., 1946; Rorschach, 1921/1951; Sarason, 1954).

4. *Hd* **responses in greater than normal number** (Phillips & Smith, 1953; Weiner, 1961a).

5. *Hd* **mouth content emphasized** (Bochner & Halpern, 1945; Schafer, 1948, 1954; Wiener, 1956).

6. *A* **responses in greater than normal number** (Beck, 1945; Bochner & Halpern, 1945; Exner, 1974; Rorschach, 1921/1951).

7. **Blood content emphasized** (Brar, 1970; Phillips & Smith, 1953; Schafer, 1948).

8. **Smoke content emphasized** (Brar, 1970; Elizur, 1949; Phillips & Smith, 1953; Schafer, 1954).

9. **Water landscape content emphasized** (Phillips & Smith, 1953).

10. **Few content categories used** (Hertz, 1948, 1949).

11. **Unpleasant or dysphoric tone to Rorschach content** (Endicott & Jortner, 1966; Hertz, 1965; Molish, 1967).

12. **Dead or dying** *H, A,* **or Plant content** (Endicott & Jortner, 1966).

13. **Dark clouds, or cold or coldness content** (Endicott & Jortner, 1966).

Other Rorschach Indices

1. **Subnormal number of** *P* **responses** (Bradway & Heisler, 1953; Goldfried et al., 1971; Weiner, 1961a).

2. **Abnormally large number of** *P* **responses** (Allison et al., 1968; Weiner, 1961a).

3. **Criticizing the Rorschach cards** (Schafer, 1948).

4. **Excessive and slow card turning behavior** (Beck, 1945).

5. **Excessive qualifications of responses** (Beck, 1945).

6. **Impotence** (Hertz, 1948).

7. **Subnormal number of responses** (Alcock, 1963; Beck, 1945; Bradway & Heisler, 1953; Brar, 1970; Hertz, 1948, 1949; Holt, 1968; Kahn & Giffen, 1960; Pope & Scott, 1967; Rorschach, 1921/1951; Schafer, 1948).

8. **Abnormally long reaction and response times** (Alcock, 1963; Allen, 1954; Allison et al., 1968; Beck, 1945; Bochner & Halpern, 1945; Harris, 1960; Hertz, 1948, 1949; Holt, 1968; Kahn & Giffen, 1960; Piotrowski, 1957; Pope & Scott, 1967; Schachtel, 1966; Schafer, 1948).

9. **Rejections or failures present** (Allen, 1954; Holt, 1968; Pope & Scott, 1967).

10. **Achromatic responses to Cards III and V** (Ames & Gillespie, 1973).

11. **Shock to Card IV** (Ames et al., 1971; Bohm, 1960, 1977; Goldfried et al., 1971; Schachtel, 1966).

12. **Shock to Card VI** (Goldfried et al., 1971; Klopfer et al., 1954; Phillips & Smith, 1953; Piotrowski, 1957).

Projective Drawing Signs

Graphological and General Indices

1. **Very small drawings** (Gurvitz, 1951; Halpern, 1965; Hammer, 1969a; Hetherington, 1952; Koppitz, 1966c; Levine & Sapolsky, 1969; Lewinsohn, 1964; Machover, 1949; Roback & Webersinn, 1966; Urban, 1963).
2. **Abnormally low placement** (Buck, 1950, 1964; Halpern, 1965; Hammer, 1954c, 1958; Jolles, 1971; Jolles & Beck, 1953b; Levy, 1950; Machover, 1949; Mursell, 1969; Urban, 1963).
3. **Abnormally light pressure** (Buck, 1964; DeCato & Wicks, 1976; Gilbert, 1969; Hammer, 1954c, 1958, 1968; Jolles, 1971; Urban, 1963).
4. **Strokes that are very short, circular, and sketchy** (Buck, 1964; Gurvitz, 1951; Hammer, 1958; Jolles, 1971; Levy, 1950, 1958; Urban, 1963).
5. **Heavy shading used, especially in agitated depressions** (Gilbert, 1969; Levine & Sapolsky, 1969; Wolk, 1969).
6. **An abnormal lack of detail** (Hammer, 1954c).
7. **Extreme bilateral symmetry in drawings** (Hammer, 1958; Modell & Potter, 1949; Urban, 1963).
8. **Lower left-hand corner placement** (Buck, 1948).

Draw-A-Person/Human Figure Drawing Indices

1. **Mouth unduly emphasized** (Gilbert, 1969; Machover, 1949; Urban, 1963).
2. **Mouth omitted** (Koppitz, 1966c; Machover, 1949; Urban, 1963).
3. **An unsmiling mouth drawn as a single line** (McElhaney, 1969).
4. **Nose unusually large or strongly reinforced** (Gilbert, 1969; Levy, 1958; Urban, 1963).
5. **Hands omitted** (Buck, 1948, 1964, 1966; DiLeo, 1973; Gilbert, 1969; Hammer, 1953a, 1958, 1960; Mundy, 1972; Schildkrout et al., 1972; Urban, 1963).
6. **Arms omitted** (Buck, 1966; DiLeo, 1973; Gilbert, 1969; Gurvitz, 1951; Halpern, 1965; Hammer, 1954c; Holzberg & Wexler, 1950; Jolles, 1969, 1971; Kahn & Giffen, 1960; Koppitz, 1966a, 1968; Levy, 1958; Machover, 1949; Urban, 1963).
7. **Resistance to drawing feet** (Machover, 1949).
8. **Beginning person drawing with legs and feet** (Levy, 1950, 1958).
9. **A stick figure is drawn for a human figure** (Gilbert, 1969).
10. **A stiff posture on person drawing** (Gilbert, 1969).
11. **Female figure is drawn much smaller than male by a male subject** (Roback & Webersinn, 1966).

H-T-P House and Tree Drawing Indices

1. **House drawn as seen from below, a worm's-eye view** (Jolles, 1971).
2. **Trees drawn as bleak or dead** (Barnouw, 1969; Buck, 1948; Hammer, 1953b, 1958; Jolles, 1969, 1971).
3. **Tree drawn in a depression** (Buck, 1964).
4. **Tree drawn as a weeping willow** (Hammer, 1969a).
5. **Tree drawn as seen from above, a bird's-eye view** (Buck, 1948, 1964; Hammer, 1954c, 1958; Jolles, 1971).
6. **Roots drawn on bottom edge of paper** (Hammer, 1958).

Bender-Gestalt Signs

1. **Curvature flattened** (DeCato & Wicks, 1976; Hutt, 1977; Hutt & Briskin, 1960).
2. **Downward sloping or mild clockwise rotation of Bender figures** (DeCato & Wicks, 1976; Halpern, 1951; Hutt, 1977; Weissman & Roth, 1965).
3. **Reversals present** (Bender, 1938).
4. **Tremors and motor incoordination** (Tucker & Spielberg, 1958).
5. **Abnormally small reproductions** (Gilbert, 1969; Hutt, 1977; Lerner, 1972).
6. **Crowded, compressed, or cohesive arrangements** (Johnson, 1973; Murray & Roberts, 1956; Pascal & Suttell, 1951; White, 1976).
7. **Figure 1 drawn with a downward slope** (Hutt, 1977; Lerner, 1972).
8. **A tiny, compressed reproduction of Figure 1** (Lerner, 1972).
9. **The horizontal direction lost with Figure 2 acquiring a curve below the initial base line** (Halpern, 1951; Hutt, 1977; Hutt & Briskin, 1960; Lerner, 1972).
10. **Figure 6 reproduced with a mild clockwise rotation and with light wavy lines** (Hutt, 1977; Hutt & Briskin, 1960).
11. **Figure 6 reproduced with a drop-off or precipitous downturning of the horizontal line** (Lerner, 1972).
12. **The crossing point on Figure 6 leaves a majority of the upright line below it** (Weissman & Roth, 1965).
13. **Figure A placed low on the page** (DeCato & Wicks, 1976).
14. **An overly methodical sequence** (Hutt, 1977).
15. **Crossing difficulty manifested** (Hutt, 1977).
16. **Sequential decrease in figure size noted** (Hutt, 1977).

Contraindication of Mania

1. **Frequent erasures on projective drawings or the Bender-Gestalt** (Ogdon, 1975).

Contraindication of Depression

1. *W+* **responses on the Rorschach** (Bochner & Halpern, 1945; Holt, 1968).

CHAPTER 5
ACTING OUT, CHARACTER, AND SEXUAL ABERRATIONS

ACTING OUT

Acting out behavior has been defined as "manifesting the purposive behavior appropriate to an older situation in a new situation which symbolically represents it" (English & English, 1958). This behavior gives overt expression to feelings and impulses. Individuals who act out may be more motivated to avoid displeasure than to gain pleasure. Such individuals are unable to move from the impulse to act to considering the consequences of impulse expression. As Fenichel (1945) put it, "They cannot perform the step from acting to thinking" (p. 507). Analysts have come to feel that strong oral fixations and early trauma are etiological factors of consequence (Alexander, 1948; Fenichel, 1945).

In his excellent chapter on the concept of acting out, Bellak (1965) indicated that acting out behavior makes "a simple unconscious statement" of conflicts and frustrated motives. These acts need not be psychopathological, although clinicians are much more sensitive to abnormal, dangerous, or illegal expressions. Psychological literature includes among acting out behavior various activities which vary from normal or near normal behavior to that which is frankly bizarre. Examples vary from overeating in the face of frustration, to phobic behavior, to acts of sexual offenders and psychopaths, paranoid psychotics acting on delusional information, and homocidal and suicidal behavior of extremely disturbed individuals.

Acting out behavior, then, ranges from essentially normal "chance actions" or "symptomatic actions" of normal individuals, as described by Freud (1904/1971) to the bizarre and grotesque acts of some psychopaths and psychotics.

Clinically significant acting out behavior falls into three general categories, two of which are related to Freud's basic instincts of death and sex, and a third, rebelliousness, added by Lindner (cf. Papanek, 1965). Death embraces intrapunitive expressions as in suicide and extrapunitive forms as in the various forms of homicide. Sexual acting out includes promiscuous heterosexual behavior, homosexuality, and sundry psychosexual deviations. Rebelliousness includes negativism and destructive behavior which is less violent than homicide or suicide—a broad range of acts from temper tantrums to stealing, setting fires, assault, etc.

In this section we follow current usage and will consider only the more extreme dangerous forms of acting out: assaultive, homicidal, and suicidal behavior. Psychological test signs of acting out behavior tendencies are presented below in three specific categories, those associated with aberrant acting out behavior in general, hostile or aggressive acting out proclivities, and finally, suicidal propensities. A presentation of contraindications of aberrant acting out concludes this section.

Subsequent sections deal, in part, with acting out behavior of delinquents, psychopaths, and sexually acting out individuals.

Test Indices for General Acting Out Behavior

Wechsler Signs
1. **PIQ significantly above VIQ** (Allison, 1978; Allison et al., 1968; Guertin et al., 1966; Hays, Solway, & Schreiner, 1978; Kaufman, 1979; Manne, Kandel, & Rosenthal, 1962; Rapaport et al., 1945; Saccuzzo & Lewandowski, 1976; Schafer, 1948; Wechsler, 1958; Wiens, Matarazzo, & Gaver, 1959; Zimmerman & Woo-Sam, 1973).
2. **Information is unusually low** (Franklin, 1945; Panton, 1960; Rabin & McKinney, 1972; Saccuzzo & Lewandowski, 1976; Zimmerman & Woo-Sam, 1973).
3. **Comprehension is unusually low** (Clark, 1948; Fisher & Sunukjian, 1950; Glasser & Zimmerman, 1967; Gurvitz, 1951; Waugh & Bush, 1971).
4. **Picture Arrangement is unusually low** (Blatt, 1965; Blatt & Quinlan, 1967; Glasser & Zimmerman, 1967; Gurvitz, 1951; Pope & Scott, 1967; Rapaport et al., 1945; Saccuzzo & Lewandowski, 1976).
5. **Arithmetic is unusually low** (Saccuzzo & Lewandowski, 1976).

Rorschach Signs
1. **High *CF*** (Adams et al., 1963; Allison et al., 1968; Ames et al., 1952, 1971; Beck, 1945, 1951, 1960; Bochner & Halpern, 1945; Klopfer et al., 1954; Levitt & Truumaa, 1972; Mons, 1950; Mundy, 1972; Munroe, 1945; Phillips & Smith, 1953; Piotrowski, 1957; Pope & Scott, 1967; Rapaport et al., 1946; Rorschach, 1921/1951; Sarason, 1954; Schachtel, 1966; Schafer, 1948, 1954; Shapiro, 1960).
2. **Numerous *CF-* responses** (Allen, 1954; Klopfer & Davidson, 1962; Phillips & Smith, 1953; Schafer, 1948; Shapiro, 1960).

3. **CF + C high and greater than FC** (Allison et al., 1968; Bochner & Halpern, 1945; Brown et al., 1961; Exner, 1969a, 1978; Haskell, 1961; Klopfer & Davidson, 1962; Korchin, 1960; Murstein, 1958, 1960; Phillips & Smith, 1953; Rorschach, 1921/1951; Rosenzweig & Kogan, 1949; Sarason, 1954; Schachtel, 1943; Shapiro, 1960; Siegal et al., 1962; Singer, 1960).

4. **CF greater than FC** (Alcock, 1963; Allison et al., 1968; Klopfer et al., 1954; Palmer, 1970; Piotrowski, 1957; Rorschach, 1921/1951; Schafer, 1948).

5. **High FM** (Adams et al., 1963; Alcock, 1963; Ames et al., 1959, 1971; Halpern, 1953; Kahn & Giffen, 1960; Klopfer & Davidson, 1962; Levitt & Truumaa, 1972; Piotrowski, 1957, 1960; Singer et al., 1956; Wagner, 1971).

6. **Unusually low M** (Cooper & Caston, 1970; Kahn, 1967; Nickerson, 1969; Perdue, 1964; Piotrowski, 1969; Singer & Herman, 1954).

7. **M% near 100** (Levi, 1965).

8. **Pure C, crude C, or Color naming responses** (Allen, 1954; Allison et al., 1968; Ames et al., 1971; Beck, 1945, 1960; Bochner & Halpern, 1945; Klopfer & Davidson, 1962; Levi, 1965; Levitt & Truumaa, 1972; Mons, 1950; Piotrowski, 1957; Rapaport et al., 1946; Rorschach, 1921/1951; Rosenzweig & Kogan, 1949; Sarason, 1954; Schachtel, 1943; Shapiro, 1960; Sommer & Sommer, 1958; Stavrianos, 1971).

9. **FC + CF + C greater than twice the number of achromatic responses (Fc + c + C')** (Hertz, 1965; Klopfer & Davidson, 1962; Piotrowski, 1957).

10. **VIII-IX-X% greater than 40** (Bochner & Halpern, 1945; Klopfer et al., 1954; Meyer, 1961; Rosenzweig & Kogan, 1949).

11. **Shock to Card II** (Hertz, 1949, 1965; Phillips & Smith, 1953; Rabin, 1946).

12. **F% greater than 50** (Adams et al., 1963; Mundy, 1972; Perdue, 1964).

13. **S locations with F- determinants** (Fonda, 1977).

Bender-Gestalt Signs

1. **Curvature exaggerated** (Billingslea, 1948; Clawson, 1959, 1962; Guertin, 1952, 1954a, 1954b; Halpern, 1951; Hutt, 1953; Hutt & Briskin, 1960; Tolor, 1968; Weiner, 1966).

2. **Making circles for dots on Figures 1 or 3** (Brown, 1965).

3. **Producing an extra loop on Figure 4** (Hutt & Briskin, 1960).

4. **Crossing point on Figure 6 leaves a majority of the horizontal line on the right** (Lerner, 1972).

5. **Lines of Figure 6 extend off the paper** (Brown, 1965).

6. **Sequential expansion of reproductions** (Brown, 1965; Clawson, 1962; Hammer, 1965, 1969b; Hutt, 1953; Hutt & Briskin, 1960; Mundy, 1972).

7. **Sequential reduction in size of reproductions** (Hutt, 1953).

Test Indices for Aggressive Acting Out Behavior

Wechsler Signs

1. **PIQ significantly greater than VIQ** (Hays et al., 1978; Manne et al., 1962; Wiens et al., 1959; Zimmerman & Woo-Sam, 1973).

2. **Unusually low Similarities score** (Kunce, Ryan, & Eckelman, 1976).

Rorschach Signs

1. **Subnormal number of M responses** (Cooper & Caston, 1970; Kahn, 1967; Nickerson, 1969; Perdue, 1964; Piotrowski, 1969; Singer & Herman, 1954), **and those given tend to be extensor M** (Schlesinger, 1978).

2. **Greater than average number of CF responses** (Beck, 1960; Exner, 1969; Finney, 1955; Rapaport et al., 1946).

3. **Pure C or crude C responses present** (Allen, 1954; Allison et al., 1968; Ames et al., 1971; Beck, 1945, 1960; Bochner & Halpern, 1945; Klopfer & Davidson, 1962; Levi, 1965; Levitt & Truumaa, 1972; Mons, 1950; Piotrowski, 1957; Rapaport et al., 1946; Rorschach, 1921/1951; Rosenzweig & Kogan, 1949; Sarason, 1954; Schachtel, 1943; Shapiro, 1960; Sommer & Sommer, 1958; Stavrianos, 1971).

4. **Color naming responses present** (Phillips & Smith, 1953).

5. **Sum C greater than three and accompanied by many CF responses** (Finney, 1955).

6. **Sum C between 1 and 3.5** (Perdue, 1964).

7. **FM greater than 2M** (Kaswan et al., 1960; Sarason, 1954).

8. **W greater than 2M** (Perdue, 1964).

9. **F% greater than 50** (Perdue, 1964).

10. **CF with aggressive content** (Klopfer et al., 1954).

11. **Confabulations, abnormal content combinations present** (Friedman, 1952; Goldfried et al., 1971; Hersch, 1962; Mons, 1950; Santostefano & Baker, 1972).

12. **Contaminations, abnormal thought combinations present** (Beck, 1945; Friedman, 1953; Goldfried et al., 1971; Hersch, 1962; Santostefano & Baker, 1972).

13. **Aggressive, hostile content in human responses** (Arnaud, 1959; Aronow & Reznikoff, 1976; Beck, 1945; DeVos, 1952; Elizur, 1949; Goldfried et al., 1971; Haskell, 1961; Kagan, 1960; Klopfer & Davidson, 1962; Piotrowski, 1977; Rader, 1957; Rapaport et al., 1946).

14. **Blood content present in significant numbers** (Allison et al., 1968; Aronow & Reznikoff, 1976; Kaswan et al., 1960; Lindner, 1947; Mons, 1950; Phillips & Smith, 1953; Rapaport et al., 1946; Stavrianos, 1971).

15. **Mutilated content present** (Arnaud, 1959; DeVos, 1952; Elizur, 1949; Goldfried et al., 1971; Rader, 1957).

16. **Explosion content emphasized** (Allen, 1954; Aronow & Reznikoff, 1976; DeVos, 1952; Halpern, 1953; Kagan, 1960; Klopfer et al., 1954; Schafer, 1954).

17. **Knife content emphasized** (Aronow & Reznikoff, 1976; DeVos, 1952; Elizur, 1949; Kagan, 1960; Kaswan et al., 1960; Phillips & Smith, 1953).

18. **War content emphasized** (Arnaud, 1959; DeVos, 1952; Elizur, 1949; Goldfried et al., 1971; Phillips & Smith, 1953; Rader, 1957).

19. **Wild or fierce animal content emphasized** (Aronow & Reznikoff, 1976; DeVos, 1952; Elizur, 1949; Klopfer & Davidson, 1962; Mundy, 1972).

20. **Head omitted from human response** (Bochner & Halpern, 1945; Due & Wright, 1945; Klopfer et al., 1954).

21. **Teeth and gum responses emphasized** (Klopfer & Davidson, 1962; Phillips & Smith, 1953; Piotrowski, 1957; Towbin, 1959).

22. **Hostile, aggressive content, especially with a chromatic determinant** (Aronow & Reznikoff, 1976; DeVos, 1952; Elizur, 1949; Sommer & Sommer, 1958).

23. **Greater than average number of animal content responses** (Perdue, 1964; Schafer, 1948).

24. **Greater than average number of anatomy content responses** (Arnaud, 1959; Murstein, 1960; Phillips & Smith, 1953; Thompson, 1965; Wagner, 1961).

25. **Space locations emphasized** (Ames et al., 1952, 1974; Beck, 1951, 1960; Bochner & Halpern, 1945; Fonda, 1960; Ingram, 1954; Klopfer et al., 1954; Mukerji, 1969).

26. **Blocking or shock to Card I or II** (Hertz, 1965; Phillips & Smith, 1953).

27. **Criticizing the inkblots** (Haskell, 1961; Kaswan et al., 1960).

28. **Rough treatment of the cards** (Klopfer et al., 1954; Towbin, 1959).

29. **Greater than normal number of inanimate movement responses** (Ames et al., 1952, 1954, 1973; DeVos, 1952; Lester, Kendra, Thisted, & Perdue, 1975).

30. **Transparency (light bulb, ice) responses noted** (Montague & Prytula, 1975).

31. **S locations emphasized** (Molish, 1967).

Note. Shading responses to chromatic areas may be contraindicative of homicidal tendencies (Lester & Perdue, 1972), as is F greater than $XF + X$ (Goldfried et al., 1971) and shock to Card IV (Phillips & Smith, 1953).

Projective Drawing Signs
Draw-A-Person Indices

1. **Extreme asymmetry in human figure drawing or HFD** (Hammer, 1965, 1969b; Koppitz, 1966c; Machover, 1949; Mundy, 1972; Urban, 1963).

2. **Unusually large heads drawn** (Gurvitz, 1951; Levy, 1950, 1958; Wysocki & Whitney, 1965; Urban, 1963).

3. **Unusually large or strongly reinforced eyes** (Deabler, 1969; Gilbert, 1969; Griffith & Peyman, 1959; Hammer, 1954c; Jacks, 1969; Kahn & Giffen, 1960; Levy, 1950, 1958; Machover, 1949, 1951, 1958; McElhaney, 1969; Reznikoff & Nicholas, 1958; Schildkrout et al., 1972; Urban, 1963).

4. **Frowning eyebrows** (McElhaney, 1969).

5. **Nose emphasized, especially with nostril indicated and emphasized** (Goldstein & Rawn, 1957; Machover, 1949; Modell & Potter, 1949; Schildkrout et al., 1972; Urban, 1963).

6. **Sharply pointed nose on HFD** (Hammer, 1965, 1969b).

7. **Teeth showing in a drawing by an adult** (Buck, 1964, 1966; Goldstein & Rawn, 1957; Halpern, 1965; Hammer, 1958, 1965; Jolles, 1971; Koppitz, 1966c, 1968; Levy, 1950, 1958; Machover, 1949, 1960; McElhaney, 1969; Reynolds, 1978; Schildkrout et al., 1972; Urban, 1963).

8. **Slash line for mouth** (Goldstein & Rawn, 1957; Levy, 1958; Machover, 1949; McElhaney, 1969; Urban, 1963).

9. **Sneering expression on lips** (McElhaney, 1969).

10. **Hair emphasized, especially with heavy shading** (Shneidman, 1958; Urban, 1963).

11. **Omission of facial features** (Machover, 1949).

12. **Chin unusually emphasized** (Buck, 1964, 1966; Jolles, 1971; Levy, 1950, 1958; Machover, 1949; McElhaney, 1969; Urban, 1963).

13. **An unusually short, thick neck** (Machover, 1949).

14. **Neck omitted** (Buck, 1964; Jolles, 1971; Koppitz, 1968; Machover, 1949; Mundy, 1972; Urban, 1963).
15. **One-dimensional neck** (Urban, 1963).
16. **Pointed shoulders** (Hammer, 1969b).
17. **Squared shoulders** (Buck, 1964, 1966; Goldstein & Rawn, 1957; Hammer, 1954c, 1958, 1965; Jolles, 1971; Urban, 1963).
18. **Massive or excessively broad shoulders drawn by males** (Hammer, 1958, 1969b; Levy, 1950; Machover, 1949).
19. **Reinforced arms, especially with emphasis on muscles and broad shoulders** (DiLeo, 1970, 1973; Hammer, 1954c, 1958, 1969b; Jolles, 1971; Machover, 1949; Shneidman, 1958).
20. **More than five fingers drawn on one hand** (Machover, 1949; Urban, 1963).
21. **Large, especially very large hands** (Buck, 1964, 1966; Jolles, 1971).
22. **Talon-like, dark straight lines, or spiked fingers** (Brown, 1958; Buck, 1964, 1966; Goldstein & Rawn, 1957; Hammer, 1954c, 1958, 1965; Jacks, 1969; Jolles, 1971; Machover, 1949; McElhaney, 1969; Reynolds, 1978; Schildkrout et al., 1972; Shneidman, 1958; Urban, 1963; Wolk, 1969).
23. **Fingers without hands, when drawn by adults, especially if drawn in one dimension with heavy pressure** (Machover, 1949; Shneidman, 1958).
24. **Fingernails emphasized or sharply pointed** (Schildkrout et al., 1972).
25. **Clenched fingers drawn as fists** (Buck, 1964; Goldstein & Rawn, 1957; Hammer, 1954c; Levy, 1950, 1958; Machover, 1949; McElhaney, 1969; Urban, 1963).
26. **Large, especially very large fingers** (Shneidman, 1958).
27. **A wide stance, particularly when the figure is placed in the middle of the page** (Buck, 1964; Hammer, 1969b; Jolles, 1971; Machover, 1949; Shneidman, 1958; Urban, 1963).
28. **Strongly reinforced legs** (Shneidman, 1958).
29. **Emphasis on feet or shoes, especially if sharply pointed** (Hammer, 1954c; Jacks, 1969; Machover, 1951, 1958; Reynolds, 1978; Schildkrout et al., 1972; Shneidman, 1958; Urban, 1963).
30. **Bare feet on an otherwise fully clad figure** (Hammer, 1969b; McElhaney, 1969).
31. **Toes drawn in a figure not intended to be nude** (Goldstein & Rawn, 1957; Machover, 1949; McElhaney, 1969; Urban, 1963).
32. **Violent action depicted in figure drawing** (Allen, 1958).
33. **Weapons drawn with the figure drawing as tucked in the belt or carried in the hand, etc.**

(Deabler, 1969; Hammer, 1965, 1969b; McElhaney, 1969; Urban, 1963).

Graphological and General Indices
1. **Very heavy pressure** (Halpern, 1951; Hammer, 1965, 1968, 1969b; Hutt, 1977; Jolles, 1971; McElhaney, 1969; Reynolds, 1978; Shneidman, 1958; Urban, 1963; Wysocki & Whitney, 1965).
2. **Unusually large drawings** (Buck, 1964; Hammer, 1954c, 1958, 1965, 1968, 1969b; Kadis, 1950; Koppitz, 1968; Levy, 1950, 1958; Machover, 1949; Precker, 1950; Urban, 1963).
3. **Placement on left side of page** (Bradfield, 1964; Buck, 1948, 1964; Hammer, 1954c, 1958, 1965, 1969a, 1969b; Jolles, 1958, 1971; Jolles & Beck, 1953a; Urban, 1963).
4. **Central placement, especially if figure is unusually large or with a wide stance** (Machover, 1949).
5. **Drawing utilizes side edge of paper** (Hammer, 1954c; Jolles, 1971).
6. **Turning paper from presented orientation** (Hammer, 1954c; Jolles, 1971).
7. **Jagged lines emphasized** (Hammer, 1965; Krout, 1950; Machover, 1951; Urban, 1963; Waehner, 1946).

House and Tree Drawing Indices
1. **H-T-P House drawn as an outhouse** (Buck, 1966; Deabler, 1969; Jacks, 1969).
2. **Enormous, page-filling drawing of House or Tree** (Buck, 1948).
3. **H-T-P Tree drawing has pointed limbs or leaves** (Hammer, 1960, 1965, 1969b; Jacks, 1969).
4. **Trees drawn leaning to the left** (Buck, 1964; Hammer, 1965; Jolles, 1971).
5. **Keyhole-type of tree drawn** (Jolles, 1971).
6. **Tree drawn with an enormous trunk** (Buck, 1964; Jolles, 1971).
7. **Tree drawn with club-like or spear-like branches** (Buck, 1964, 1966; Hammer, 1954c, 1958, 1969b; Jacks, 1969; Jolles, 1971; Mursell, 1969).
8. **Tree drawn with branches thickening to the outside** (Koch, 1952).
9. **Tree drawn with talon-like roots** (Buck, 1964, 1966; Hammer, 1954c; Jolles, 1971).
10. **Tree drawn with a dog or other animal urinating on it** (Deabler, 1969; Hammer, 1954c; Jacks, 1969).

Bender-Gestalt Signs
(See above under Graphological and General Indices of acting out for signs for possible use with the Bender-Gestalt.)

1. **Collision arrangements** (Brown, 1965; Clawson, 1962; DeCato & Wicks, 1976; Halpern, 1951; Hutt & Briskin, 1960; Hutt & Gibby, 1970).
2. **Scattered, expansive arrangements** (Clawson, 1959, 1962; DeCato & Wicks, 1976; Halpern, 1951; Hutt & Briskin, 1960; Hutt & Gibby, 1970).
3. **Requiring several sheets of paper for the Bender reproductions** (Brown, 1965; Clawson, 1962).
4. **Very large reproductions** (Brown, 1965; Clawson, 1962; Halpern, 1951; Haworth & Rabin, 1960; Hutt, 1977; Mundy, 1972; Palmer, 1970; Tolor, 1968).
5. **Sequential expansion of reproductions** (Brannigan & Benowitz, 1975; Brown, 1965; Clawson, 1962; Hammer, 1965, 1969b; Hutt, 1953, 1977, 1978; Hutt & Briskin, 1960; Mundy, 1972).
6. **Closure difficulty** (Brown, 1965; Halpern, 1951).
7. **Flattened curvature** (Hutt & Briskin, 1960).
8. **Turning design card or paper** (Clawson, 1962; Haworth & Rabin, 1960).
9. **Overlapping and crossing difficulty** (Brown, 1965; Halpern, 1951; Hutt & Gibby, 1970).
10. **On Figure 1, heavily slashed dashes substituted for dots** (Brown, 1965; DeCato & Wicks, 1976; Lerner, 1972).
11. **On Figure 4, overlapping of parts** (Brown, 1965; Lerner, 1972; Weissman & Roth, 1965).
12. **On Figure 5, lines substituted for dots** (Halpern, 1951; Lerner, 1972).
13. **On Figure 5, dashes or circles substituted for dots** (Brown, 1965).
14. **On Figure 6, angles, straight lines, or spikes produced in the curves** (Brown, 1965; DeCato & Wicks, 1976).
15. **On Figure 7, points elongated with slashing lines** (Lerner, 1972).
16. **Sequential reduction in size of figures** (Hutt, 1953).
17. **Exaggerated curvature** (Brannigan & Benowitz, 1975).
18. **Uneven figure size** (Brannigan & Benowitz, 1975).
19. **Counterclockwise rotations** (DeCato & Wicks, 1976).

Test Indices for Suicidal Acting Out Propensities

Wechsler Signs
1. **Unusually low Arithmetic score** (Levenson, 1974; Levenson & Neuringer, 1971).
2. **Unusually low Digit Symbol score** (Henrichs & Amolsch, 1978).
3. **Unusually low Block Design** (Henrichs & Amolsch, 1978).
4. **Unusually low Object Assembly score** (Henrichs & Amolsch, 1978).
5. **Unusually high Comprehension score** (Henrichs & Amolsch, 1978).
6. **Unusually high Vocabulary score** (Henrichs & Amolsch, 1978).
7. **VIQ significantly greater than PIQ** (Henrichs & Amolsch, 1978).

Rorschach Signs
Determinant and Location Indices
1. *CF or C* response first occurs to Plate VIII, IX, or X; this has been considered one of the best single Rorschach signs of suicide potential (Cutter et al., 1968; Daston & Sakheim, 1960; Goldfried et al., 1971; Neuringer, 1974; Weiner, 1961a).
2. **Surface shading responses to chromatic areas** (Appelbaum & Colson, 1968; Appelbaum & Holzman, 1962; Colson & Hurwitz, 1973; Exner, 1978; Exner & Wylie, 1977; Goldfried et al., 1971; Hertz, 1965; Weiner, 1977).
3. **Subnormal number of *CF* responses, particularly between zero and three** (Cutter et al., 1968; Daston & Sakheim, 1960; Goldfried et al., 1971; Neuringer, 1974; Weiner, 1961a).
4. *FC + CF + C* **is approximately zero** (Cerbus & Nichols, 1963; Hertz, 1965; Weiner, 1961a).
5. **Sum *C* between 1 and 3.5** (Cerbus & Nichols, 1963; Cutter et al., 1968; Daston & Sakheim, 1960; Goldfried et al., 1971; Neuringer, 1974; Rapaport et al., 1946; Weiner, 1961a).
6. *CF + C* **+ Sum of Shading responses equals zero** (Cutter et al., 1968).
7. **Pure *C* or crude *C* responses present, especially if they first appear to Plates VIII, IX, or X** (Kendra, 1979; Neuringer, 1974; Weiner, 1961a; White & Schreiber, 1952).
8. **No achromatic responses given** (Neuringer, 1974; Weiner, 1961a), **or presence of black color responses** (Exner, 1974; Kendra, 1979; Piotrowski, 1977).
9. **Sum of Achromatic + Texture responses equals zero** (Daston & Sakheim, 1960; Neuringer, 1974).
10. *FC + CF + C* **greater than twice** *Fc + c + C'* (Hertz, 1965).
11. *Fm + m* **greater than** *M + FM* (Hertz, 1965; White & Schreiber, 1952).
12. **Sum *C* approximately equals *M* and both are near zero** (Beck, 1960; Gurvitz, 1951; Neuringer, 1974; Palmer & Lustgarten, 1962; Rapaport et

al., 1946; Rickers-Ovsiankina, 1960; Rorschach, 1921/1951; Schafer, 1948; Weiner, 1961a).

13. *CF* + *C* **greater than** *FC* (Exner, 1978; Exner & Wylie, 1977).

14. **Greater than average number of surface shading responses** (Hertz, 1965; White & Schreiber, 1952).

15. **No surface shading or Vista responses given** (Goldfried et al., 1971; Neuringer, 1974; Weiner, 1961a).

16. *F%* **greater than 60 with** *P* **less than 3** (Neuringer, 1974; Weiner, 1961a).

17. *M* **or** *FM* **with hostile content** (Hertz, 1965; Piotrowski, 1957), **or with joyful, pleasant, or dancing content** (Piotrowski, 1977).

18. *M* **with** *S* **locations** (Bohm, 1958; Hertz, 1965), **or with animal content** (Sakheim, 1955).

19. *S* **greater than 3** (Exner, 1978; Exner & Wylie 1977).

20. **An unusual number of** *D* **locations used: less than 6 or greater than 20** (Alcock, 1963; Beck, 1945; Neuringer, 1974; Weiner, 1961a).

21. *3r* + (2)/*R* **is less than .3** (Exner, 1978; Exner & Wylie, 1977).

22. **Greater than normal number of Vista responses, with or without the use of shading** (Exner, 1974).

Content and Other Rorschach Indices

1. **Greater than average number of** *Hd* **responses** (Neuringer, 1974; Phillips & Smith, 1953; Weiner, 1961a).

2. *H* **less than 2, especially if zero** (Exner, 1978; Exner & Wylie, 1977).

3. **Map content emphasized** (Costello, 1958; Phillips & Smith, 1953).

4. **Weird or bizarre content such as deformed or moribund** *A* **or** *H* **content** (Hertz, 1965; Piotrowski, 1977).

5. **Subnormal number of Popular responses** (Bradway & Heisler, 1953; Exner, 1978; Exner & Wylie, 1977; Goldfried et al., 1971; Neuringer, 1974; Weiner, 1961a).

6. **Greater than average number of Popular responses** (Allison et al., 1968; Exner, 1978; Exner & Wylie, 1977; Kendra, 1979; Neuringer, 1974; Weiner, 1961a).

7. **Blocking or shock to Card I** (Hertz, 1965; Phillips & Smith, 1953; Schafer, 1954).

8. **Blocking or shock to Card II** (Hertz, 1965; Rabin, 1946).

9. **Blocking or shock to Card IV** (Hertz, 1965; Rabin, 1946; Sakheim, 1955).

10. **Deteriorating or dysphoric content to Card IV** (Broida, 1954; Cutter et al., 1968; Hertz, 1965; Lindner, 1947, 1950).

11. **Blocking or shock to Card VI** (Goldfried et al., 1971; Klopfer et al., 1954; Phillips & Smith, 1953; Piotrowski, 1957).

12. **VIII-IX-X% less than 30** (Weiner, 1961a).

13. **Any response given to the bottom center** *D* **of Card VII, Beck's D6** (Hertz, 1965; Goldfried et al., 1971; Sapolsky, 1963).

14. **An unusually high** *F%* (Alcock, 1963; Allison et al., 1968; Bohm, 1958; Goldfried et al., 1971; Hertz, 1965; Levitt & Truumaa, 1972).

15. **Transparency (e.g., light bulb), translucency (e.g., ice), and cross-section (e.g., X-ray) responses emphasized** (Blatt & Ritzler, 1974; Rierdan, Lang, & Eddy, 1978).

16. *R* **less than 17,** *H* **less than 2, and** *S* **greater than 3** (Exner, 1978; Exner & Wylie, 1977).

17. **Pleasant, tranquil, joyful responses** (Beck, 1978; Piotrowski, 1977).

Projective Drawing Signs

1. **Omission of arms on DAP** (Buck, 1966; DiLeo, 1973; Gurvitz, 1951; Halpern, 1965; Hammer, 1954c; Holzberg & Wexler, 1950; Jolles, 1969, 1971; Kahn & Giffen, 1960; Kokonis, 1972; Koppitz, 1966b, 1968; Levy, 1958; Machover, 1949; Mursell, 1969; Urban, 1963).

2. **Slash lines on DAP body, even though they appear inadvertent** (Schildkrout et al., 1972).

3. **H-T-P Tree drawn dead** (Barnouw, 1969; Buck, 1948; Hammer, 1958; Jolles, 1969, 1971).

4. **H-T-P Tree drawn with thick, very short "cut off" branches** (Brown cited in Buck, 1964; Buck, 1966).

Bender-Gestalt Signs

1. **On Figure 6, a drop-off or precipitous downturning of the horizontal line** (Lerner, 1972).

2. **When sinusoidal curves of Figure 6 penetrate the space of Figure 5** (DeCato & Wicks, 1976; Eisenthal, 1974; Sternberg & Levine, 1965).

Contraindications

Rorschach Signs

1. *M* **greater than twice** *FM* (Klopfer et al., 1954; Meyer, 1961).

2. *M* **greater than** *FM* **with** *FM* **equal to one or zero** (Klopfer et al., 1954; Meyer, 1961).

3. **Greater than average number of achromatic responses** (Phillips & Smith, 1953).

4. **Abstract content emphasized** (Phillips & Smith, 1953).

5. **Greater than average number of anatomy responses** (Phillips & Smith, 1953; Rapaport et al., 1946).

6. **Surface shading responses to chromatic areas are contraindicative of aggressive acting out** (Lester & Perdue, 1972).

7. *FC* **greater than** *CF* + *C* (Klopfer et al., 1954).

PSYCHOPATHY, SOCIOPATHY, AND DELINQUENCY

Test Indices

Wechsler Signs

1. **Performance IQ significantly above the Verbal IQ** (Allison, 1978; Allison et al., 1968; Altus & Clark, 1949; Bernstein & Corsini, 1953; Blank, 1958; Diller, 1952; Franklin, 1945; Gilbert, 1969; Glueck & Glueck, 1964; Graham & Kamano, 1958; Guertin et al., 1966; Harris, 1957; Kaufman, 1979; Lewandowski, Saccuzzo, & Lewandowski, 1977; Manne et al., 1962; Rapaport et al., 1945; Saccuzzo & Lewandowski, 1976; Schafer, 1948; Sloan & Cutts, 1945; Wechsler, 1958; Wiens et al., 1959; Zimmerman & Woo-Sam, 1973).

2. **Performance IQ normal with the Verbal IQ subnormal** (Prentice & Kelly, 1963).

3. **Unusually low Information scores** (Franklin, 1945; Lewandowski et al., 1977; Panton, 1960; Rabin & McKinney, 1972; Saccuzzo & Lewandowski, 1976; Zimmerman & Woo-Sam, 1973).

4. **Unusually low Arithmetic scores** (Altus & Clark, 1949; Franklin, 1945; Lewandowski et al., 1977; Rabin & McKinney, 1972; Saccuzzo & Lewandowski, 1976; Schafer, 1948; Sloan & Cutts, 1945; Strother, 1944; Zimmerman & Woo-Sam, 1973).

5. **Unusually high Digit Span scores** (Allison et al., 1968; Schafer, 1948).

6. **Unusually low Comprehension scores** (Gilbert, 1969; Harris, 1957; Lewandowski et al., 1977; Schafer, 1948; Zimmerman & Woo-Sam, 1973).

7. **Unusually high Comprehension scores** (Gilbert, 1969; Holt, 1968; Wittenborn & Holzberg, 1951).

8. **Unusually high Similarities scores** (Lewandowski et al., 1977; Wittenborn & Holzberg, 1951).

9. **Unusually low Similarities scores with PIQ significantly above the VIQ and an unusually high Picture Arrangement score** (Schafer, 1948).

10. **Unusually high Picture Arrangement scores** (Allison et al., 1968; Blank, 1958; Foster, 1959; Franklin, 1945; Gilbert, 1969; Graham & Kamano, 1958; Patterson, 1953; Saccuzzo & Lewandowski, 1976; Schafer, 1948; Wechsler, 1958; Wittenborn & Holzberg, 1951; Zimmerman & Woo-Sam, 1973).

11. **Unusually high Picture Completion scores** (Franklin, 1945; Schafer, 1948; Wittenborn & Holzberg, 1951; Zimmerman & Woo-Sam, 1973).

12. **Unusually high Object Assembly scores** (Altus & Clark, 1949; Blank, 1958; Franklin, 1945; Sloan & Cutts, 1945; Zimmerman & Woo-Sam, 1973).

13. **Unusually low Block Design scores** (Foster, 1959; Franklin, 1945; Zimmerman & Woo-Sam, 1973).

Rorschach Signs

1. *M* + *FM* **is equal to or less than 1** (Klopfer & Davidson, 1962).

2. **Pure** *C* **responses are present** (Beck, 1945; Exner, 1969; Shapiro, 1977; Rorschach, 1921/1951).

3. *F%* **is less than 20** (Schafer, 1948).

4. **An abnormally high number of animal responses present** (Perdue, 1964; Schafer, 1948).

5. **Visceral or soft anatomy responses emphasized** (Phillips & Smith, 1953).

6. **Blood content emphasized** (Allison et al., 1968; Kaswan et al., 1960; Lindner, 1947; Mons, 1950; Phillips & Smith, 1953; Rapaport et al., 1946; Stavrianos, 1971).

7. **Knife content emphasized** (Elizur, 1949; Kagan, 1960; Kaswan et al., 1960; Phillips & Smith, 1953).

8. **Map and geography content emphasized** (Halpern, 1953; Kahn & Giffen, 1960; Klopfer & Davidson, 1962; Phillips & Smith, 1953).

9. **Nature and landscape content emphasized** (Ames et al., 1952; Bochner & Halpern, 1945).

10. **Reflection content emphasized** (Bochner & Halpern, 1945; Exner, 1969, 1974).

11. **War content emphasized, especially with fighting and** *M* **determinants** (Phillips & Smith, 1953; Schafer, 1954).

12. **Rejections or failures manifested** (Bochner & Halpern, 1945; Prandoni, Jensen, Matranga, & Waison, 1973).

13. **Rough treatment of Rorschach cards noted** (Klopfer et al., 1954).

14. **A subnormal number of responses** (Schafer, 1948).

15. *DW* **responses are emphasized** (Alcock, 1963; Piotrowski, 1957; Schafer, 1948).

16. **A void of** *cF* **responses** (Schafer, 1948).

17. **Transparency (e.g., light bulb, ice) responses emphasized** (Montague & Prytula, 1975).
18. **Primitive, aggressive content emphasized** (Harrow et al., 1976).

Projective Drawing Signs
Graphological and General Signs
1. **Very heavy pressure used** (Hammer, 1958).
2. **A very large drawing made** (Machover, 1949; McElhaney, 1969; Urban, 1963).
3. **Shading never used** (Deabler, 1969).

Draw-A-Person/Human Figure Drawing Signs
1. **Back of a person is drawn** (Allen, 1958).
2. **A clown, soldier, or witch is drawn** (Levy, 1950; Urban, 1963).
3. **A cowboy is drawn** (Deabler, 1969; Urban, 1963).
4. **A stick figure is drawn** (Buck, 1964; Deabler, 1969; Hammer, 1969a; Jolles, 1971; Urban, 1963).
5. **A wide stance is drawn** (Machover, 1949).
6. **Overclothed figures, especially if drawn energetically by a female** (Machover, 1949).
7. **Pockets emphasized** (Levy, 1958; Machover, 1949, 1958; Urban, 1963).
8. **Genitalia drawn** (Deabler, 1969; DiLeo, 1973).
9. **Weapons drawn tucked in the belt or carried in the hand** (Deabler, 1969; Gilbert, 1969; Hammer, 1965, 1969b; McElhaney, 1969).
10. **Hands drawn behind the back, out of sight** (McElhaney, 1969).
11. **Clenched fingers made into fists** (Buck, 1964; Goldstein & Rawn, 1957; Hammer, 1954c; Levy, 1950, 1958; Machover, 1949; McElhaney, 1969; Urban, 1963).
12. **Hands drawn in pockets** (DiLeo, 1973; Jolles, 1971; Machover, 1949; McElhaney, 1969; Schildkrout et al., 1972; Urban, 1963).

H-T-P House Drawing Signs
1. **An outhouse drawn** (Buck, 1966; Deabler, 1969; Jacks, 1969).

Bender-Gestalt Signs
Unusual Reproduction Modes and Arrangements
1. **Closure difficulty noted** (Brown, 1965; Halpern, 1951).
2. **Dots changed to circles** (Gilbert, 1969).
3. **Unusually large reproductions made** (Gilbert, 1969; Halpern, 1951).
4. **Perseveration manifested** (Halpern, 1951).

5. **Regression, including simplification, primitivation, or condensation manifested** (Halpern, 1951).
6. **Tremors and motor incoordination noted** (Curnutt, 1953; Hutt, 1953; Pascal & Suttell, 1951; Zolik, 1958).
7. **A scattered, expansive arrangement made** (Halpern, 1951).
8. **Numerous sheets of paper required for this test** (Brown, 1965; Clawson, 1962).

Unusual Treatment of Specific Figures
1. **Figure A placed in the center of the page** (Clawson, 1962; Hutt, 1953, 1968), **or in lower corner** (Hutt, 1977).
2. **Straight lines used to portray dots on Figure 1** (Halpern, 1951).
3. **Dashes used for dots on Figure 3** (Bender, 1938; Burgemeister, 1962; Halpern, 1951; Zolik, 1958).
4. **Lines substituted for dots on Figure 5** (Halpern, 1951; Lerner, 1972).
5. **Asymmetry of contour manifested on Figure 6** (Zolik, 1958).
6. **Extra angles drawn on Figure 7** (Zolik, 1958).

Contraindication of Psychopathy
1. **Rorschach *M* responses associated with abstract content** (Phillips & Smith, 1953).

PSYCHOSEXUAL DISTURBANCES

Freud (1905/1938) classified sexual deviations into two major categories: deviations of sexual object and deviations of sexual aim. Psychodiagnostic research has been sparse regarding most of these deviations, and it is not appropriate to try to cover all of them in this volume. We generally subscribe to the point of view that an individual does not have a psychosexual deviation as long as his or her primary mode of achieving sexual gratification is through sexual intercourse with an adult member of the opposite sex. Individuals with such an appropriate sex object who engage in sundry sexual activities which are essentially precursory sexual aims should not be considered sexually deviant. Examples of such behavior which may be considered as more or less appropriate sexual foreplay include exhibitionistic, voyeuristic, and other related activities which usually include some kind of genital contact. As long as these are not the person's primary mode of sexual gratification we would not consider them deviant and we would not expect them to manifest the psychological signs noted below.

Furthermore, a person who rarely engages in homosexual behavior, a deviation of sex object, particularly if this occurs when appropriate sex objects are not available, may not be expected to display psychological manifestations associated with individuals who are largely or exclusively homosexual.

Most of the diagnostic research in this area has focused on male homosexuality. A smaller number of studies have dealt with female homosexuality and a very few with other sexually abnormal conditions. This should be kept in mind when using the psychological signs noted below. Further, studies dealing with narcissism and exhibitionism more often have dealt with these tendencies in individuals near the normal end of these dimensions. Thus the test signs regarding them as outlined below do not necessarily point to obvious sexually maladjusting conditions.

Whether or not sexually deviant individuals should be considered abnormal is a concept given a good deal of current consideration, though such a discussion is beyond the scope of this work. Criteria used to consider them abnormal are twofold and broadly comparable with those that define most functional aberrations. The majority of our society apparently regards them as abnormal, and statistically they are not normal. Obviously no organic deficit or biological deviation is necessarily implied.

The following list of test indices has three parts. The first deals with sexual disturbances and conflicts in general. Included here are test signs associated with protocols of sex offenders as well as those of individuals with clinically significant sexual conflicts and other functional sexual disturbances. The second part deals specifically with homosexuality. The third covers narcissism and exhibitionism which, in the extreme, have been considered a deviation of sexual object and a deviation of sexual aim, respectively. They are considered together here because our literature review revealed that they share many test signs, and often they appear to be psychodynamically related as well.

Test Indices of General Psychosexual Disturbances

Rorschach Signs

1. **Sex content emphasized** (Allen, 1954; Andersen & Seitz, 1969; Armon, 1960; Beck, 1945; Bochner & Halpern, 1945; Brar, 1970; Due & Wright, 1945; Klopfer & Davidson, 1962; Mukerji, 1969; Phillips & Smith, 1953; Piotrowski, 1957; Schafer, 1954).
2. **Water or landscape content emphasized** (Phillips & Smith, 1953; Piotrowski, 1957).
3. **Tree and leaf types of content emphasized** (Phillips & Smith, 1953; Piotrowski, 1957).
4. **Genitalia content present** (Brar, 1970; Klopfer & Davidson, 1962; Wheeler, 1949).
5. **Rejections or failures manifested** (Bochner & Halpern, 1945; Prandoni et al., 1973).
6. **Shock noted to Card II** (Bohm, 1958; Coates, 1962; Piotrowski, 1957).
7. **Shock noted to Card III** (Phillips & Smith, 1953; Piotrowski, 1957).
8. **Blocking or shock to Card IV** (Klopfer et al., 1954; Phillips & Smith, 1953; Piotrowski, 1957).
9. **A limp penis response given to upper outer detail on Card IV** (McCully, 1971).
10. **Blocking or shock to Card VI** (Allen, 1954; Ames et al., 1971; Brown, 1963; Klopfer et al., 1954; Meyer, 1961; Mundy, 1972; Phillips & Smith, 1953; Piotrowski, 1957; Pope & Scott, 1967; Prandoni et al., 1973).

Projective Drawing Signs
Person Drawing Signs
1. **Opposite sex is drawn first** (Allen, 1958; Armon, 1960; Barnouw, 1969; Green, Fuller, & Rutley, 1972; Hammer, 1954c; Jolles, 1971; Kurtzberg, Cavior, & Lipton, 1966; Laird, 1962; Levy, 1950, 1958; Machover, 1949, 1951; McElhaney, 1969; Pollitt et al., 1964; Urban, 1963; Wysocki & Wysocki, 1977).
2. **Hair omitted or drawn inadequately** (Buck, 1950; Hammer, 1953a).
3. **Eyebrows drawn with considerable elaboration by males, especially if very trim or arched in style** (Hammer, 1968; Urban, 1963).
4. **Nose drawn unusually large, long, or strongly reinforced** (Buck, 1964, 1966; DiLeo, 1973; Hammer, 1953a, 1954c; Jolles, 1971; Machover, 1949; Wysocki & Wysocki, 1977).
5. **Mouth a slash line or emphasized by males** (Jolles, 1971; Machover, 1949; Urban, 1963; Wysocki & Wysocki, 1977).
6. **Full lips drawn on male figure by a male** (Geil, 1944; Hammer, 1968; Levy, 1950; Machover, 1949; Urban, 1963).
7. **Rounded trunks drawn** (Gurvitz, 1951; Levy, 1950; Machover, 1949).
8. **Reluctance to close the bottom of the trunk** (Jolles, 1971; Machover, 1949; Urban, 1963).
9. **A heavy line or other excessive emphasis noted at the waist** (Buck, 1964, 1966; Hammer, 1954c; Jolles, 1971; Machover, 1949; Wysocki & Wysocki, 1977).

10. **Waistline drawn unusually high or low** (Machover, 1949).

11. **Waist area is excessively shaded** (Buck, 1964, 1966; Jolles, 1971).

12. **Hands drawn so as to cover the genital region** (Buck, 1964, 1966; Hammer, 1954c; Jolles, 1971; Machover, 1949; Urban, 1963).

13. **Buttocks emphasized** (Buck, 1964, 1966; DiLeo, 1973; Geil, 1944; Hammer, 1954c, 1968; Jolles, 1971; Levy, 1950; Machover, 1949; Urban, 1963).

14. **Legs drawn pressed closely together** (Buck, 1964; Jolles, 1969, 1971; Schildkrout et al., 1972; Urban, 1963).

15. **Muscular legs on female figures or feminine legs drawn on male figures** (Machover, 1949).

16. **Feet drawn with excessive emphasis or length** (Hammer, 1954c; Machover, 1951, 1958; Schildkrout et al., 1972; Shneidman, 1958; Urban, 1963; Wysocki & Wysocki, 1977).

17. **Refusal to draw the human figure below the waist** (Buck, 1966; Jolles, 1971; Kokonis, 1972; Machover, 1949; Urban, 1963).

18. **Males draw the female figure larger, more muscular, or with a wide stance while same sex figure is puny** (Levy, 1958; McElhaney, 1969; Pollitt et al., 1964).

19. **An unusually large or distorted head drawn** (Wysocki & Wysocki, 1977).

Person's Clothing and Miscellaneous
Appurtenance Signs

1. **Overclothed figures, especially when drawn with significant energy** (Levy, 1950, 1958; Machover, 1949).

2. **An underclothed or nude figure drawn** (Gurvitz, 1951; Jolles, 1971; Levy, 1950, 1958; Machover, 1949; Schildkrout et al., 1972; Urban, 1963).

3. **Transparent clothing drawn** (Machover, 1949).

4. **Elaborate or emphasized belts** (Buck, 1964, 1966; Gilbert, 1969; Jolles, 1971; Machover, 1949; Urban, 1963).

5. **Trouser fly is emphasized** (McElhaney, 1969).

6. **Tie emphasized by reinforcement, length, or conspicuousness** (Buck, 1964, 1966; Hammer, 1954c; Jolles, 1971; Levy, 1950, 1958; Machover, 1949; Schildkrout et al., 1972; Urban, 1963).

7. **Tiny, uncertainly drawn, or debilitated ties drawn** (Levy, 1958; Machover, 1949).

8. **Tie drawn as blown off to one side** (Machover, 1949; Urban, 1963).

9. **Pipe drawn very large, conspicuous, or actively smoked** (Levy, 1950, 1958; Machover, 1949, 1951).

10. **Figure drawn with cigarette, cane, or gun** (Buck, 1964; Levy, 1950, 1958; Machover, 1949, 1951; Urban, 1963).

H-T-P House and Tree Drawing Signs

1. **Multiple chimneys drawn** (Hammer, 1954c; Jolles, 1971).

2. **Chimney emphasized by reinforcement or size** (Buck, 1948, 1964, 1966; Hammer, 1953a, 1954c; Jolles, 1969, 1971; Landisberg, 1969; Mursell, 1969).

3. **A phallic Tree drawn** (Allen, 1958; Jolles, 1952b, 1971).

Bender-Gestalt Signs

1. **On Figure 6, excessive erasure, inability to complete crossing, and upright lines extending only partially through the horizontal one** (Hammer, 1954b).

2. **On Figure 8, drawing either point open** (Weissman & Roth, 1965).

3. **On Figure 7, the hexagonal figures are drawn shortened or with rounded ends** (Hutt, 1977).

4. **On Figure 8, difficulty in reproducing the extremities or changing the size of the diamond** (Hutt, 1977).

Test Indices of Homosexual Tendencies

Rorschach Signs

Determinant Signs

1. *M* responses with *(H)* content (Phillips & Smith, 1953).

2. **Greater than normal number of inanimate movement responses** (Phillips & Smith, 1953).

3. *FC + CF + C* approximates zero (Armon, 1960).

4. **Reflection (*Fr + rF*) responses given** (Exner, 1974).

5. **Numerous pair (2) responses given** (Exner, 1974). 1974).

Content Signs

1. **Sex identification of *H* content is confused, evasive, or vacillating** (Andersen & Seitz, 1969; Due & Wright, 1945; Fine, 1950; Klopfer & Davidson, 1962; Lindner, 1946, 1947, 1950; Miale, 1947; Phillips & Smith, 1953; Piotrowski, 1957; Reitzell, 1949; Schafer, 1954).

2. **Humans seen back to back** (Aronow & Reznikoff, 1976; Goldfried, 1966a; Goldfried et al., 1971; Hooker, 1958; Kwawer, 1977; Reitzell, 1949; Stone & Schneider, 1975; Weiner, 1977; Wheeler, 1949; Yamahiro & Griffith, 1960).

3. *(H)* responses present in significant number, especially witches or monsters to Card IX, D3, and humanized animals, e.g., Bugs Bunny to Card V (Due & Wright, 1945; Klopfer & Davidson, 1962; Kwawer, 1977; Piotrowski, 1957; Wheeler, 1949).

4. Unusual *Hd* content with the head omitted from human responses (Bochner & Halpern, 1945; Due & Wright, 1945; Klopfer et al., 1954).

5. *AH* responses given (Armon, 1960; Kwawer, 1977; Wheeler, 1949).

6. Eye content emphasized, especially if "peering" or "piercing" (Alcock, 1963; Allen, 1954; Beck, 1960; Bochner & Halpern, 1945; Bradway & Heisler, 1953; Due & Wright, 1945; Fonda, 1960; Kahn & Giffen, 1960; Klopfer et al., 1954; Lindner, 1946, 1947; Phillips & Smith, 1953; Piotrowski, 1957; Pope & Scott, 1967; Reitzell, 1949).

7. Oral detail given, especially when concomitant with anal detail (Andersen & Seitz, 1969; Armon, 1960; Aronson, 1952; DeLuca, 1966; Goldfried, 1966b; Hooker, 1958; Kwawer, 1977; Reitzell, 1949; Schafer, 1948, 1954; Stone & Schneider, 1975; Weiner, 1977; Wheeler, 1949; Yamahiro & Griffith, 1960).

8. Anal or buttocks content given in significant number (Andersen & Seitz, 1969; Aronow & Reznikoff, 1976; Aronson, 1952; Brar, 1970; Davids, Joelson, & McArthur, 1956; Goldfried, 1966b; Goldfried et al., 1971; Hooker, 1958; Kwawer, 1977; Lindner, 1946, 1947, 1950; Miale, 1947; Phillips & Smith, 1953; Piotrowski, 1957; Reitzell, 1949; Schafer, 1948, 1954; Stone & Schneider, 1975; Weiner, 1977; Wheeler, 1949).

9. Genitalia content present (Aronow & Reznikoff, 1976; Brar, 1970; Davids et al., 1956; DeLuca, 1966; Klopfer & Davidson, 1962; Kwawer, 1977; Reitzell, 1949; Stone & Schneider, 1975; Weiner, 1977; Wheeler, 1949; Yamahiro & Griffith, 1960).

10. Anatomy responses present in greater than normal number (Due & Wright, 1945).

11. Feminine clothing emphasized by males (Andersen & Seitz, 1969; Aronow & Reznikoff, 1976; Aronson, 1952; Due & Wright, 1945; Fine, 1950; Goldfried, 1966b; Goldfried et al., 1971; Halpern, 1953; Hooker, 1958; Klopfer et al., 1954; Kwawer, 1977; Piotrowski, 1957; Reitzell, 1949; Schafer, 1954; Stone & Schneider, 1975; Weiner, 1977; Wheeler, 1949; Yamahiro & Griffith, 1960).

12. Mask content emphasized (Due & Wright, 1945; Kwawer, 1977; Reitzell, 1949; Wheeler, 1949).

13. Animals seen back to back (Aronow & Rezni-koff, 1976; Goldfried, 1966; Goldfried et al., 1971; Hooker, 1958; Kwawer, 1977; Piotrowski, 1957; Reitzell, 1949; Stone & Schneider, 1975; Weiner, 1977; Wheeler, 1949; Yamahiro & Griffith, 1960).

14. Art and design content emphasized by men (Phillips & Smith, 1953; Piotrowski, 1957).

15. Mutilated or deformed content present (Andersen & Seitz, 1969; Aronow & Reznikoff, 1976; Due & Wright, 1945).

16. Frightening, aggressive, or Amazon female figures given, particularly by females (Andersen & Seitz, 1969; Armon, 1960; Aronow & Reznikoff, 1976; Schafer, 1954).

17. Religious content, objects, activities, etc. (Aronson, 1952; Kwawer, 1977; Reitzell, 1949; Stone & Schneider, 1975; Weiner, 1977; Wheeler, 1949; Yamahiro & Griffith, 1960).

18. Ambiguous sex organ content (Aronow & Reznikoff, 1976).

19. Household furniture content emphasized (Reitzell, 1949).

Other Rorschach Indices

1. On Card I, the human form in center *D* is seen as a male by a male (Aronow & Reznikoff, 1976; Aronson, 1952; DeLuca, 1966; Kwawer, 1977; Lindner, 1950; Reitzell, 1949; Weiner, 1977; Wheeler, 1949; Yamahiro & Griffith, 1960).

2. Shock manifested to Card III by males (Phillips & Smith, 1953; Piotrowski, 1957).

3. On Card III, confusion, uncertainty, or difficulty noted in determining the sex of the popular *H* (Aronson, 1952; Kwawer, 1977; Lindner, 1950; Reitzell, 1949; Weiner, 1977; Wheeler, 1949), or identifying the *H* as bisexual (Aronow & Reznikoff, 1976).

4. On Card III, a *W* or cut off *W*, seen as *A* or dehumanized animal-like content (Aronson, 1952; DeLuca, 1966; Reitzell, 1949; Weiner, 1977; Wheeler, 1949; Yamahiro & Griffith, 1960).

5. Card IV seen as a monstrous, threatening figure by a male (Aronow & Reznikoff, 1976; Aronson, 1952; Davids et al., 1956; Goldfried, 1966b; Goldfried et al., 1971; Kwawer, 1977; Reitzell, 1949; Stone & Schneider, 1975; Weiner, 1977; Wheeler, 1949; Yamahiro & Griffith, 1960).

6. Card V seen by males as human or humanized animal content (Aronow & Reznikoff, 1976; Davids et al., 1956; DeLuca, 1966; Goldfried, 1966b; Goldfried et al., 1971; Kwawer, 1977; Reitzell, 1949; Stone & Schneider, 1975; Weiner, 1977; Wheeler, 1949; Yamahiro & Griffith, 1960).

7. **Card VII seen by males as depreciated female content,** e.g., "old bag" (Aronow & Reznikoff, 1976; Aronson, 1952; Davids et al., 1956; Goldfried, 1966b; Goldfried et al., 1971; Kwawer, 1977; Reitzell, 1949; Stone & Schneider, 1975; Weiner, 1977; Wheeler, 1949; Yamahiro & Griffith, 1960).

8. **On Card VIII, the lateral *D* described as an animal with incongruous parts of several incongruous animals** (Aronson, 1952; Reitzell, 1949; Weiner, 1977; Wheeler, 1949; Yamahiro & Griffith, 1960).

9. **On Card IX, the upper lateral described as a dehumanized *H* (a witch or monster)** (Aronson, 1952; Reitzell, 1949; Stone & Schneider, 1975; Weiner, 1977; Wheeler, 1949; Yamahiro & Griffith, 1960).

10. **On Card X, the top central *D* described as animals being aggressive toward the central object** (Aronson, 1952; Kwawer, 1977; Reitzell, 1949; Weiner, 1977; Wheeler, 1949; Yamahiro & Griffith, 1960).

11. **On Card X, *H* content with blue detail reported as an oral specification** (Reitzell, 1949; Wheeler, 1949).

Projective Drawing Signs

Draw-A-Person/Human Figure Drawing Signs

1. **Opposite sex is drawn first** (Allen, 1958; Armon, 1960; Barnouw, 1969; Geil, 1944; Green et al., 1972; Hammer, 1954c; Jolles, 1971; Kurtzberg et al., 1966; Levy, 1950, 1958; Machover, 1949, 1951; McElhaney, 1969; Pollitt et al., 1964; Urban, 1963; Wysocki & Wysocki, 1977).

2. **Hair emphasized, especially when vigorously shaded** (Levy, 1950, 1958).

3. **Eyebrows drawn with considerable elaboration or emphasis by males** (Hammer, 1968; Urban, 1963).

4. **Eyelashes detailed by males** (DeMartino, 1954; DiLeo, 1973; Geil, 1944; Machover, 1949; Urban, 1963).

5. **Unusually large or strongly reinforced eyes drawn by males** (Geil, 1944; Levy, 1950, 1958; Machover, 1949; Urban, 1963).

6. **Ears drawn unusually large or strongly reinforced** (DiLeo, 1973; Levy, 1958; Machover, 1949; Urban, 1963).

7. **Full lips on male figure drawn by a male** (Geil, 1944; Hammer, 1968; Levy, 1950; Machover, 1949; Urban, 1963).

8. **A wasp waist in a male's drawing of a male** (Levy, 1950, 1958).

9. **Rounded trunks drawn** (Gurvitz, 1951; Levy, 1950; Machover, 1949).

10. **Reluctance to close the bottom of the trunk** (Jolles, 1971).

11. **Buttocks emphasized** (Buck, 1964, 1966; DiLeo, 1973; Geil, 1944; Hammer, 1954c, 1968; Jolles, 1971; Levy, 1950; Machover, 1949; Urban, 1963).

12. **A male figure drawn twisted in perspective to emphasize hips and buttocks** (Geil, 1944; Machover, 1949).

13. **Hips emphasized in drawings by males** (DiLeo, 1973; Geil, 1944; Hammer, 1968; Levy, 1950; Machover, 1949, 1951; Urban, 1963).

14. **Knees emphasized** (Buck, 1964, 1966; Hammer, 1954c; Jolles, 1971; Schildkrout et al., 1972; Urban, 1963).

15. **Nose emphasis through pressure or size** (DiLeo, 1973; Machover, 1949).

Person's Clothing and Miscellaneous Appurtenance Signs

1. **Transparent pants drawn to reveal legs** (Machover, 1949).

2. **Boots drawn on male figures by males** (McElhaney, 1969).

3. **Shoes emphasized with high heels detailed by or on male figure drawn by a male** (DeMartino, 1954; Hammer, 1968; Urban, 1963).

4. **Males drawing male figures with canes** (McElhaney, 1969).

5. **Human figure drawn scantily clad, nude, or with emphasis on breasts or genital area** (Hassell & Smith, 1975).

Bender-Gestalt Signs

1. **Overlapping and crossing difficulty manifested** (Billingslea, 1948; Hutt & Gibby, 1970).

2. **On Figure 7, elongated deviations noted** (Halpern, 1951; Hutt, 1953; Hutt & Briskin, 1960).

3. **On Figure 7, overlapping difficulty** (Billingslea, 1948; Hutt, 1968).

4. **On Figures 7 and 8, closure difficulty manifested** (Buck, 1968).

5. **On Figure 8, a disturbance of elongation noted** (Halpern, 1951).

6. **Subparts of Figure 7 are overlapping with longitudinal axes parallel** (DeCato & Wicks, 1976).

Test Indices of Narcissism and Exhibition

Wechsler Signs

1. **Unusually low Arithmetic scores** (Allison et al., 1968; Blatt & Allison, 1968).

2. **PIQ significantly above VIQ** (Zimmerman & Woo-Sam, 1973).

Rorschach Signs

1. **Abnormally high number of CF responses given** (Exner, 1969a).
2. **CF + C unusually high and greater than number of FC** (Allison et al., 1968; Brown et al., 1961; Exner, 1969a; Phillips & Smith, 1953; Rorschach, 1921/1951; Rosenzweig & Kogan, 1949; Sarason, 1954; Shapiro, 1960, 1977).
3. **CF with S responses present** (Schafer, 1954).
4. **Pure C responses manifested** (Beck, 1945; Exner, 1969a; Rorschach, 1921/1951).
5. **A subnormal number of Fc responses noted** (Klopfer & Davidson, 1962; Meyer, 1961; Munroe, 1945).
6. **A greater than average number of shading responses given** (Mukerji, 1969).
7. **Shock to Card III present** (Phillips & Smith, 1953; Piotrowski, 1957).
8. **Reflection content emphasized** (Ames et al., 1959, 1971; Bochner & Halpern, 1945; Exner, 1969a, 1974).
9. **By females, an abnormally large number of clothing responses** (Phillips & Smith, 1953; Piotrowski, 1957; Schafer, 1954).
10. **Pair (2) responses emphasized** (Exner, 1974).

Projective Drawing Signs

Draw-A-Person/Human Figure Drawing Signs

1. **The same sex figure drawn with considerable neatness and elaboration while opposite sex is smaller and dilapidated** (Gilbert, 1969).
2. **Seductive figures drawn by females** (McElhaney, 1969).
3. **Transparent clothing drawn** (Deabler, 1969; Machover, 1949).
4. **An underclothed or nude figure drawn** (Gurvitz, 1951; Jolles, 1971; Levy, 1950, 1958; Machover, 1949; Schildkrout et al., 1972; Urban, 1963).
5. **A front view of an overdressed figure is drawn** (Levy, 1950, 1958; Machover, 1949, 1951; Urban, 1963).
6. **The drawing is begun with measurement details or use of props for bilateral control** (Machover, 1949).
7. **A clown is drawn** (Urban, 1963).
8. **A profile of the head is drawn with the body in a front view** (Machover, 1949; Urban, 1963).
9. **An unusually large head drawn** (Machover, 1949, 1951; Urban, 1963).
10. **Hair significantly emphasized** (Buck, 1964; Levy, 1950, 1958; Machover, 1949; McElhaney, 1969; Urban, 1963).

11. **Males draw hair carefully and precisely on male figure and messily on the female figure** (Machover, 1949, 1951; Urban, 1963).
12. **Unusually large or strongly reinforced eyes drawn** (Machover, 1951; Urban, 1963).
13. **Long, phallic noses drawn** (Hammer, 1969b).
14. **Full lips on a male figure drawn by a male** (Hammer, 1968; Levy, 1950; Machover, 1949; Urban, 1963).
15. **Earrings emphasized** (Jolles, 1971; Levy, 1950, 1958).
16. **Unusually large breasts drawn by a female** (Buck, 1966; McElhaney, 1969).
17. **Joints emphasized** (Hammer, 1968; Kahn & Giffen, 1960; Machover, 1949, 1951; Urban, 1963).
18. **Overdetailing of feet** (Buck, 1966; Jolles, 1971; Urban, 1963).
19. **Arms drawn akimbo** (Machover, 1949).
20. **Excessively tight waistline** (Machover, 1949, 1958; Urban, 1963).

H-T-P House and Tree Drawing Signs

1. **Chimney emphasized through size or reinforcement** (Buck, 1948, 1966; Hammer, 1969a; Jolles, 1971; Levine & Sapolsky, 1969; Mursell, 1969).
2. **An unusually large number of windows drawn** (Buck, 1948).
3. **An enormous tree drawn on an arc-like hill or well centered** (Buck, 1948, 1964, 1966; Jolles, 1971; Levine & Sapolsky, 1969).
4. **A tree drawn that is rugged and large and isolated on a hilltop** (Buck, 1948, 1964, 1966; Jolles, 1971).
5. **Trees drawn leaning to the left** (Koch, 1952).

Bender-Gestalt Signs

1. **Figure 1 placed in the the center of the page** (Clawson, 1962; DeCato & Wicks, 1976; Hutt, 1953, 1968, 1977, 1978).
2. **Figure A centrally placed with the other figures drawn encircling it** (Hutt, 1977; Hutt & Briskin, 1960).
3. **Angulation changed on Figure 1 so the whole design describes an arc** (Hutt, 1977; Hutt & Briskin, 1960).
4. **Angulation changed on Figure 2 so the whole design describes an arc** (Hutt, 1968, 1977; Hutt & Briskin, 1960).
5. **Figure 6 drawn with exaggerated amplitude of the curves** (Weissman & Roth, 1965).

CHAPTER 6
ORGANICITY

The aim here is to provide information for diagnosing damage to the central nervous system from a "standard battery" of psychological tests. Beyond this, data are also provided to generate hypotheses regarding the site of the damage when it is either lateralized to the left or right hemisphere or focalized in a particular lobe or other identifiable areas of the brain.

In 1937, Zigmunt Piotrowski published his classic paper on the Rorschach technique with organic, brain-damaged patients. He presented both behavioral and Rorschach indices which tended to separate brain-damaged from functional psychiatric patients. In the 1940s, Halstead (1947) followed with his neuropsychological test battery to refine the process of distinguishing between brain-damaged and non-brain-damaged persons. Through the next quarter of a century Reitan (1962, 1964, 1967, 1974), Luria (1963, 1964), McFie (1960, 1975), and Russell, Neuringer, and Goldstein (1970), among others, worked to further the study of brain-behavior relationships, to improve diagnosing brain damage, and, with varying degrees of success, to localize the cite of the damage if it was not diffuse. These clinicians primarily used tests and subtests of intelligence, reasoning, concept formation, and perceptual-motor abilities. Most of Piotrowski's signs have stood the test of time reasonably well as far as screening patients who are brain-damaged from patients who are not (Ogdon, 1975). Difficulty sometimes arises in attempting differential diagnoses between schizophrenia and organicity. The effectiveness of psychological test batteries to identify organicity, as well as specific sites of central nervous system damage, continues to be evaluated (cf. McFie, 1975; Small, 1973; Smith & Philippus, 1969). As McFie (1975) optimistically noted, "Further neuropsychological research will undoubtedly identify with greater precision those cognitive abilities which are mediated by specific parts of the brain" (p. 149).

Specialists in neuropsychological diagnosis tend to employ batteries of various psychological, psychoeducational, and other tests. For example, Reitan uses 10 to 13 tests (Reitan & Davison, 1974), while McFie (1975) uses three tests (a Wechsler scale plus tests of auditory and visual memory). Boll (1978) has concluded, "If one's goal is strictly diagnosis, it is quite likely that neither the battery of tests nor the [protracted] training period need be so long" (p. 66). Allison (1978) seems to agree with McFie (1975) who stated, "With the conclusion of the Wechsler subtests, the major abilities whose impairment may suggest a cerebral lesion have been sampled, with the exception . . . of memory" (pp. 24–25). Others have developed "short forms" of the extensive Halstead-Reitan battery (Erickson, Calsyn, & Scheupbach, 1978; Golden, 1976). More elaborate and comprehensive test batteries are likely to lead to significant contributions to our understanding of behavioral correlates of normal and abnormal brain functions. On the other hand, a clinician who uses a typical assessment battery, such as the tests included in this volume, may do essentially as well in developing diagnostic impressions as the specialist with a dozen or more test instruments. Even Reitan's comprehensive battery frequently fails to distinguish between organics and functional psychotics (Lacks, Harrow, Colbert, & Levine, 1970; Watson, Thomas, Andersen, & Felling, 1968), though the Rorschach test often provides signs for such a differential diagnosis (Ogdon, 1975).

In another study, the Bender-Gestalt test "was found to be as effective as a screening measure of organicity as was the lengthy Halstead-Reitan battery" (Levine & Feirstein, 1972, p. 511). On the other hand, Hammer (1978) contended that "the H-T-P . . . is superior to the Bender-Gestalt for detecting organicity" (p. 298). He also quoted a personal communication from Landisberg declaring, "Evidence of organicity is discerned in a more clear-cut fashion with the H-T-P than with the Rorschach" (p. 298).

DeWolfe et al. (1971) reported data that suggest that differential diagnoses between organic and psychiatric patients made on a basis of Wechsler subtest scores are comparable to or as good as those made from a complete set of Halstead-Reitan scores. Experts in this area are not of one mind. The value of the Halstead-Reitan battery in localizing the site of a lesion continues to be evaluated.

This chapter reviews neuropsychological literature from the point of view that diagnoses of organicity, and reasonable hypotheses concerning the site of localized brain damage, can be obtained from a standard battery of clinical, psychological tests, though a more extensive, specialized battery may be appropriate for difficult cases and for research purposes.

Wechsler subtests least affected by brain damage and therefore expected to be relatively high in test profiles of organics, include Vocabulary (Lezak, 1976; McFie, 1960; Overall, Hoffman, & Levin, 1978), Information (Lezak, 1976; Overall et al., 1978), Comprehension (Overall et al., 1978), and Picture Completion

(McFie, 1960; Russell, 1979), although this latter sub-test may be low in test profiles of alcoholics, some of whom are brain-damaged (Hirt & Cook, 1962; O'Leary, Donovan, Chaney, Walker, & Shau, 1979; Pope & Scott, 1967). Other Wechsler subtests tend to be differentially and adversely affected by various lesion sites.

Research in neuropsychology is remarkably difficult and complex. In studying the psychological effects of localized brain damage in humans, multiple factors must be considered other than the site of the lesion. Included among these are possible effects of cerebral edema, vascular involvement, cerebral dominance or handedness, age, sex and health of the patient, age of the damage or lesion, type of lesion, whether the damage is static or not, the post-operative interval for examination, intracranial tension, etiology of the damage, amount of cerebral damage, radiating effects to the opposite hemisphere, effects of medications, and differential premorbid functioning of the individuals studied. Too often many of these potentially significant independent variables are unknown or unknowable.

Patients with a damaged left hemisphere clearly tend to do relatively poorly on verbal-linguistic tasks and manifest a VIQ below their PIQ. A VIQ significantly below the PIQ in an organic setting is a strong sign of localized left hemisphere damage. On the other hand, a PIQ significantly below the VIQ suggests the possibility of right hemisphere damage, but this is a relatively weak sign. Diffuse brain damage affects both verbal and performance functioning, although it appears to affect nonverbal, performance functioning more. Patients with diffuse and right hemisphere damage often appear similar on the Wechsler (and other neuro-psychological tests). Differential diagnosis between patients with right hemisphere damage and those with diffuse damage is much more difficult than distinguishing either of them from patients with left cerebral hemisphere damage (see signs and symptoms delineated below).

Obviously, to consider organicity as a single entity is a gross oversimplification. Nevertheless, neuropsychology appears to provide "promise for some of the most significant developments in psychological assessment and in applied psychology in general" (Maloney & Ward, 1976, p. 277). This may be correct despite Allison's (1978) caution that "efforts to develop systematic correlations of the loci of neurological damage with specific psychological dysfunction are also still in their early stages, and the known correlations may not be readily applicable to the bulk of test referrals which are likely to stem from neurological ambiguity" (p. 377). It may now be possible for the psychologist to "tell the neurologist whether or not a patient's performance resembles that of typical cases of lesion in one of the major cerebral lobes; and the neurologist can combine this information with evidence from other procedures in arriving at [the] assessment" (McFie, 1960, p. 391).

A word on the simulation of organicity is appropriate here. Bender herself addressed the topic of malingering in her original monograph (1938). More recent evidence supports the proposition that normals are not able to simulate organicity on the Bender-Gestalt. Bruhn and Reed (1975) have demonstrated that college students faking organicity and organic patients can be distinguished by a clinical psychologist (though objective Pascal-Suttell scores failed to make the distinction).

The remainder of this chapter has five parts, the first of which deals with hard and soft behavioral signs of damage to the central nervous system. Second, there are Wechsler, Rorschach, projective drawing, and Bender-Gestalt signs associated with organic conditions to aid in differential diagnosis of these conditions from normals and individuals with functional disorders. Then, test signs are presented which are useful for hypothesizing in which hemisphere localized brain damage occurs once the presence of organic dysfunctioning is ascertained. Fourth, there is an enumeration of test signs associated with focalized damage to certain lobes of the brain. This is followed by a summary of contraindications of organicity.

Behavioral Manifestations

Following are enumerations of "hard" and "soft" behavioral signs of brain damage. Such categorization is to some extent artificial, and obviously does not do justice to qualitatively different manifestations that occur with reference to a particular sign. Furthermore, not all hard signs are equally dependable. For example, aphasia and apraxia (depending on the definitions used) may not be as reliable or valid signs as pathological reflexes. Comparable differences unquestionably exist among the soft signs. Hard and soft signs of organicity have been discussed in greater detail by Lezak (1976), Luria (1963), and Small (1973). Neither type of sign will necessarily be manifested. A brain-damaged condition can exist for decades without medical significance or any recognized behavioral effect (Boll, 1978).

Hard behavioral manifestations of organicity include:
1. Pathological reflexes.
2. Unilateral movement disorders.
3. Aphasia, a loss or severe impairment of language ability.
4. Apraxia, an inability to carry out purposeful movements.

Soft behavioral manifestations of organicity include:
1. Speech disturbances, slurred, or incoherent speech.
2. Hyperkinesis, hyperactivity, easy distractibility.
3. Failure to maintain balance.
4. Disturbances of gait, awkwardness.
5. Coordination deficiencies, tremors, clumsiness.
6. Fainting or falling associated with dizziness or drowsiness.
7. Irritability or anger easily aroused.
8. Easy fatigability.
9. Dysphasia.
10. Automatic behavior.

Behavioral manifestations associated with *localized or focalized brain damage* include:
1. **Left hemisphere damage associated with auditory memory deficit** (Benton, 1967), **and forgetting what to do in given situations or circumstances** (Andersen, 1951), **with expressive and receptive language disorders** (Boll, 1978; McFie, 1975; Russell et al., 1970), **and failure in abstraction** (McFie, 1975).
2. **Right hemisphere damage associated with visual (nonverbal) memory deficit** (Benton, 1967; Boll, 1978), **and forgetting how to do what one wants to do** (Andersen, 1951).
3. **Temporo-occipital damage with dysgraphia** (Hutt, 1977; Luria, 1964), **particularly if the damage is in the left hemisphere** (Boll, 1978).
4. **Parietal-occipital area damage with impaired visual-spatial and perceptual ability** (Hutt, 1977).
5. **Parieto-temporo-occipital area damage with dyscalculia and spatial-perceptual problems** (Luria, 1964), **particularly if the damage is in the left hemisphere** (Boll, 1978).
6. **Parietal area damage with visual-spatial orientation and perceptual disturbances as well as acalculia** (Hutt, 1977).
7. **Right parietal lobe damage has been associated with apraxia and misrecognition of familiar faces** (Boll, 1978), **as well as acalculia** (McFie, 1960, 1975).
8. **Left parietal damage with aphasia, constructional apraxia, as well as acalculia** (Hutt, 1977; McFie, 1975).
9. **Right temporal lobe damage has been associated with impaired recognition of nonverbal sounds, e.g., music, noises, etc.** (Boll, 1978).
10. **Left temporal lobe damage with verbal skills, including vocabulary, impaired** (Hutt, 1977; McFie, 1975).

11. **Frontal lobe damaged patients may perform satisfactorily on structured tests with clear instructions but do poorly on other tests such as the Rorschach** (Boll, 1978); **these patients may also manifest recent memory loss, perseverative behavior, impaired ability to correct mistakes, incoordination, impaired judgment, planning ability, and visual searching or scanning behavior** (Hutt, 1977).

Finally, it should be noted that Bellak and Fielding (1978) suggested, "Anytime very poor impulse control and relatively intact thinking are found, possibly combined with a history of asocial behavior, the patient should be carefully examined for evidence of minimal brain damage" (p. 769). Thorough neurological and neuropsychological examinations should be made for a dependable diagnosis.

Test Indices

Wechsler Signs
1. **Verbal IQ significantly greater than the Performance IQ** (Allen, 1947, 1948a, 1948b; Allison, 1978; Allison et al., 1968; Balthazar & Morrison, 1961; Balthazar, Todd, Morrison, & Ziebell, 1961; Beck and Lam, 1955; Blatt & Allison, 1968; Bruell & Albee, 1962; Davis, Becker, & DeWolfe, 1971; Davison, 1974; Dennerll, 1964; DiLeo, 1973; Fisher, 1960; K.B. Fitzhugh & L.C. Fitzhugh, 1964; Fitzhugh, Fitzhugh, & Reitan, 1962; Goldfarb, 1961; Guertin et al., 1966; Heaton et al., 1979; Hirt & Cook, 1962; Hutt, 1977; Karlin, Eisenson, Hirschenfang, & Miller, 1959; Kaspar & Schulman, 1972; Klove & Fitzhugh, 1962; Kohn & Dennis, 1974; Ladd, 1964; Maloney & Ward, 1976; Morrow & Mark, 1955; Philippus, 1969; Pope & Scott, 1967; Rabin & McKinney, 1972; Reed & Reitan, 1963; Russell, 1979; Simpson & Vega, 1971; Sinnett & Mayman, 1960; Small, 1973; Smith, 1962; Smith, 1969; Smith & Smith, 1977; Wechsler, 1958; Zimmerman, Whitmyre, & Fields, 1970; Zimmerman & Woo-Sam, 1973).
2. **Unusually low Block Design score** (Aita, Armitage, Reitan, & Rabinowitz, 1947; Allen, 1947, 1948a, 1948b; Allison, 1978; Allison et al., 1968; Anthony, Heaton, & Lehman, 1980; Balthazar, 1963; Balthazar et al., 1961; Bendien, 1957; Black, 1976; Burgemeister, 1962; Davis et al., 1971; Erickson et al., 1978; Fitzhugh et al., 1962; Glasser & Zimmerman, 1967; Gonen, 1970; Greenblatt, Goldman, & Coon, 1946; Guertin

et al., 1966; Heaton et al., 1979; Heilbrun, 1959; Hirt & Cook, 1962; Holland et al., 1979; Holland & Watson, 1980; Kahn & Giffen, 1960; Levi, Oppenheim, & Wechsler, 1945; Lezak, 1976; Maloney & Ward, 1976; Matthews, Shaw, & Klove, 1966; Morrow & Mark, 1955; O'Leary et al., 1979; Parker, 1957; Parsons, Morris, & Denny, 1963; Patterson, 1953; Philippus, 1969; Pope & Scott, 1967; Rappaport, 1953; Reitan, 1955a, 1964; Russell, 1979; Russell et al., 1970; Sattler, 1974; Small, 1973; Smith, 1962; Smith & Smith, 1977; Symmes & Rapaport, 1972; Waugh & Bush, 1971; Wechsler, 1958; Zimmerman et al., 1970; Zimmerman & Woo-Sam, 1973).

3. **Unusually low Digit Symbol score** (Aita, Armitage, Reitan, & Rabinowitz, 1947; Allen, 1947, 1948a, 1948b; Allison, 1978; Anthony et al., 1980; Balthazar, 1963; Davison, 1974; Erickson et al., 1978; L.C. Fitzhugh & K. Fitzhugh, 1964; Glasser & Zimmerman, 1967; Gonen, 1970; Guertin et al., 1966; Gurvitz, 1951; Heaton et al., 1979; Hewson, 1949; Hirt & Cook, 1962; Holland et al., 1979; Holland & Watson, 1980; Hopkins, 1964; Jordan, 1970; Kaspar & Schulman, 1972; Ladd, 1964; Levi et al., 1945; Levine & Feirstein, 1972; Magaret, 1942; Maloney & Ward, 1976; Matthews et al., 1966; McFie, 1975; Morrow & Mark, 1955; O'Leary et al., 1979; Overall et al., 1978; Philippus, 1969; Pope & Scott, 1967; Reitan, 1955c; Reitan & Reed, 1962; Russell, 1972, 1979; Russell et al., 1970; Simpson & Vega, 1971; Small, 1973; Smith, 1962; Smith & Smith, 1977; Stevens, Boydstun, Dykman, Peters, & Sinton, 1967; Wechsler, 1958; Zimmerman et al., 1970; Zimmerman & Woo-Sam, 1973).

4. **Unusually low Object Assembly score** (Allen, 1947, 1948a; Allison, 1978; Anthony et al., 1980; Black, 1976; Guertin et al., 1966; Heaton et al., 1979; Holland et al., 1979; Holland & Watson, 1980; Lezak, 1976; Matthews et al., 1966; O'Leary et al., 1979; Russell, 1979; Sattler, 1974; Schafer, 1948; Simpson & Vega, 1971; Smith & Smith, 1977; Wechsler, 1958; Zimmerman et al., 1970).

5. **Unusually low Picture Arrangement score** (Aita, Armitage, Reitan, & Rabinowitz, 1947; Anthony et al., 1980; Fitzhugh et al., 1962; Greenblatt et al., 1946; Heilbrun, 1959; Hewson, 1949; Hirt & Cook, 1962; Holland et al., 1979; Holland & Watson, 1980; Lezak, 1976; Matthews et al., 1966; McFie, 1960, 1975; O'Leary et al., 1979; Patterson, 1953; Russell, 1979; Simpson & Vega, 1971; Smith & Smith, 1977; Wechsler, 1958; Zimmerman et al., 1970).

6. **Unusually low Digit Span score** (Allen, 1947, 1948a, 1948b; Blatt & Allison, 1968; Dennerll, Broeder, & Sokolov, 1964; DeWolfe, 1971; DeWolfe et al., 1971; Evans & Marmorston, 1963; Fisher, 1958; Glasser & Zimmerman, 1967; Gonen, 1970; Heaton, Smith, Lehman, & Vogt, 1978; Heaton et al., 1979; Heilbrun, 1958; Hewson, 1949; Holland et al., 1979; Holland & Watson, 1980; Kaspar & Schulman, 1972; Kove, 1959; Levi et al., 1945; Levine & Feirstein, 1972; Lezak, 1976; McFie, 1960; Morrow & Mark, 1955; Pope & Scott, 1967; Reitan, 1955c; Reitan & Reed, 1962; Russell, 1972; Russell et al., 1970; Small, 1973; Stevens et al., 1967; Tolor, 1956, 1958; Wechsler, 1958; Zimmerman & Woo-Sam, 1973).

7. **Significantly more Digits Forward than Digits Backward** (Evans & Marmorston, 1963; Holt, 1968; Lezak, 1976; Morrow & Mark, 1955).

8. **Unusually low Arithmetic score** (Aita, Armitage, Reitan, & Rabinowitz, 1947; Hewson, 1949; Hopkins, 1964; Kaspar & Schulman, 1972; Levi et al., 1945; Magaret, 1942; McFie, 1960; Morrow & Mark, 1955; O'Leary et al., 1979; Overall et al., 1978; Small, 1973; Smith, 1969; Zimmerman & Woo-Sam, 1973).

9. **Low Arithmetic with high Digit Span score** (Allison et al., 1968).

10. **Unusually low Similarities score** (Allison, 1978; Allison et al., 1968; Blatt & Allison, 1968; Benton & Howell, 1941; Fisher, 1958; Lewinski, 1947; Lezak, 1976; McFie, 1960; Milberg, Greiffenstein, Lewis, & Rourke, 1980; Morrow & Mark, 1955; Overall & Gorham, 1972; Philippus, 1969; Reitan, 1964; Russell et al., 1970; Sattler, 1974; Small, 1973; Zimmerman & Woo-Sam, 1973), **especially with many "don't know" responses** (Lezak, 1976).

11. **Unusually low Information score** (Fitzhugh et al., 1962; Kaspar & Schulman, 1972; Overall & Gorham, 1972; Rappaport, 1953; Stevens et al., 1967; Wechsler, 1958).

12. **Unusually low Picture Completion score** (Black, 1976; Hirt & Cook, 1962; Lezak, 1976).

13. **Unusually low Comprehension score** (Fitzhugh et al., 1962; Jordan, 1970; Smith, 1969), **especially with difficulty on proverb items** (Allison, 1978).

14. **Unusually low Vocabulary score** (Evans & Marmorston, 1963; Jackson, 1955), **though also seen with relatively high Vocabulary scores** (Zimmerman & Woo-Sam, 1973).

15. **Digit Span significantly below Comprehension and Vocabulary differentially diagnoses brain damage from schizophrenia** (DeWolfe, 1971; DeWolfe et al., 1971).

Rorschach Signs
Determinant Indices

1. **Subnormal number of *M* responses** (Alcock, 1963; Bohm, 1958; Evans & Marmorston, 1963; Goldfried et al., 1971; Harrower-Erickson, 1941; Hughes, 1948, 1950; Kahn & Giffen, 1960; Kisker, 1944; Klopfer et al., 1954; Neiger et al., 1962; Oberholzer cited in Kisker, 1944; Phillips & Smith, 1953; Piotrowski, 1937b, 1960, 1977; Reitan, 1955c; Ross & Ross, 1944; Weiner, 1966, 1977).

2. **Poor quality *F* responses** (Allen, 1954; Beck, 1945, 1968; Beck et al., 1961; Birch & Diller, 1959; Evans & Marmorston, 1963, 1964; Gottlieb & Parsons, 1960; Halpern, 1953; Harrower-Erickson, 1941; Kahn & Giffen, 1960; Kisker, 1944; Korchin, 1960; Neiger et al., 1962; Oberholzer cited in Kisker, 1944; Piotrowski, 1937b; Reitan, 1955c; Ross & Ross, 1944; Small, 1973; Weiner, 1966, 1977).

3. **Subnormal number of *FC* responses** (Beck, 1945; Hughes, 1948, 1950).

4. **Color naming responses present** (Alcock, 1963; Allen, 1954; Allison et al., 1968; Baker, 1956; Beck, 1945; Bohm, 1958; Brar, 1970; Halpern, 1953; Hughes, 1948, 1950; Kahn & Giffen, 1960; Molish, 1967; Neiger et al., 1962; Piotrowski, 1937b, 1957; Ross & Ross, 1944; Schachtel, 1966; Weiner, 1966).

5. **Pure *C* responses present** (Beck, 1945; Klopfer et al., 1954; Rorschach, 1921/1951; Shapiro, 1960; Werner, 1945).

6. ***CF* present in significantly greater number than *FC*** (Evans & Marmorston, 1963; Weiner, 1977).

7. ***FC + CF + C* approximately equal to zero** (Harrower-Erickson, 1941; Kisker, 1944; Reitan, 1955c; Shapiro, 1960; Smith, 1969).

8. **Subnormal number of shading responses, especially a void of shading responses** (Hertz & Loehrke, 1954).

9. **Abnormally large number of pure *c* responses** (Alcock, 1963; Klopfer et al., 1954).

10. **Few or no Vista responses** (Reitan, 1955c).

11. ***F%* greater than 80** (Philippus, 1969; Smith, 1969).

Location and Content Indices

1. ***W-* or vague *W* responses present in significant number** (Beck, 1944; Bohm, 1958; Goldfried et al., 1971; Gottlieb & Parsons, 1960; Oberholzer cited in Kisker, 1944; Sarason, 1954; Weiner, 1966).

2. **Subnormal number of *W* responses** (Goldfried et al., 1971; Piotrowski & Berg, 1955; Piotrowski & Lewis, 1950; Rorschach, 1921/1951).

3. ***DW* responses present** (Bochner & Halpern, 1945; Exner, 1974; Oberholzer cited in Kisker, 1944; Rorschach, 1921/1951).

4. **Subnormal number of *D* responses** (Reitan, 1955c).

5. ***D-* responses present** (Goldfried et al., 1971).

6. **Many *d* responses with few *W* responses** (Piotrowski, 1957).

7. ***Dd + dr + S* equal to zero** (Evans & Marmorston, 1963, 1964; Weiner, 1977; Werner, 1945).

8. ***do* responses present** (Allen, 1954; Allison et al., 1968; Werner, 1945).

9. ***Hdx* or *Adx* content present** (Klopfer et al., 1954; Lezak, 1976; Phillips & Smith, 1953; Shaw & Cruickshank, 1957; Werner, 1945).

10. **Abnormally large number of *A* responses** (Allen, 1954; Beck, 1945; Evans & Marmorston, 1963; Goldfried et al., 1971; Kral & Dorken, 1953; Oberholzer cited in Kisker, 1944; Weiner, 1977).

11. **Few content categories used** (Allison et al., 1968; Evans & Marmorston, 1963; Olch, 1971; Piotrowski & Bricklin, 1961; Sherman, 1955; Weiner, 1977).

12. **"Ink blot" for a response** (Lezak, 1976).

Other Rorschach Indices

1. **Subnormal number of *P*** (Alcock, 1963; Birch & Diller, 1959; Bohm, 1958; Goldfried et al., 1971; Kahn & Giffen, 1960; Olch, 1971; Piotrowski, 1937b; Reitan, 1955c; Shaw & Cruickshank, 1957; Small, 1973; Weiner, 1966).

2. **Subnormal number of *O*** (Beck, 1951).

3. **Subnormal number of responses** (Alcock, 1963; Allen, 1954; Ames et al., 1954, 1973; Bradway & Heisler, 1953; Evans & Marmorston, 1963; Goldfried et al., 1971; Harrower-Erickson, 1941; Hertz & Loehrke, 1954; Hughes, 1948, 1950; Kahn & Giffen, 1960; Kisker, 1944; Kral & Dorken, 1953; Lezak, 1976; Neiger et al., 1962; Philippus, 1969; Piotrowski, 1937b, 1957; Reitan, 1955c; Ross & Ross, 1944; Weiner, 1977).

4. **Abnormally long reaction and response times** (Alcock, 1963; Allen, 1954; Beck, 1945; Birch &

Diller, 1959; Goldfried et al., 1971; Kahn & Giffen, 1960; Kisker, 1944; Lezak, 1976; Neiger et al., 1962; Oberholzer cited in Kisker, 1944; Piotrowski, 1937b).

5. **Automatic phrasing used** (Goldfried et al., 1971; Lezak, 1976; Piotrowski, 1937b, 1957; Ross & Ross, 1944; Small, 1973; Weiner, 1966).

6. **Confabulations, abnormal content combinations present** (Klopfer et al., 1954; Lezak, 1976; Phillips & Smith, 1953).

7. **Contaminations, abnormal thought combinations present** (Beck et al., 1961; Goldfried et al., 1971; Hughes, 1948, 1950).

8. **Covering part of the ink blot while responding** (Aita, Reitan, & Ruth, 1947; Baker, 1956; Halpern, 1953; Klopfer et al., 1954).

9. **Edging manifested** (Aita, Reitan, & Ruth, 1947).

10. **Impotence, an inability to improve on responses recognized as inferior or inadequate** (Alcock, 1963; Allison, 1978; Baker, 1956; Beck, 1960; Birch & Diller, 1959; Evans & Marmorston, 1963; Goldfried et al., 1971; Hertz & Loehrke, 1954; Hughes, 1948, 1950; Kahn & Giffen, 1960; Luria, 1963; Mabry, 1964; Piotrowski, 1937b; Reitan, 1955c; Rosenzweig & Kogan, 1949; Ross & Ross, 1944; Small, 1973; Weiner, 1977).

11. **Perplexity, distrust of one's own ability** (Alcock, 1963; Baker, 1956; Beck, 1960; Birch & Diller, 1959; Evans & Marmorston, 1963, 1964; Goldfried et al., 1971; Hertz & Loehrke, 1954; Hughes, 1948, 1950; Kahn & Giffen, 1960; Kisker, 1944; Lezak, 1976; Neiger et al., 1962; Piotrowski, 1937b, 1957; Pope & Scott, 1967; Reitan, 1955c; Rosenzweig & Kogan, 1949; Ross & Ross, 1944; Small, 1973; Weiner, 1977).

12. **Perseverations or repetitions present** (Alcock, 1963; Allison, 1978; Baker, 1956; Beck, 1945, 1960; Bohm, 1958; Birch & Diller, 1959; Halpern, 1953; Hertz & Loehrke, 1954; Hughes, 1948, 1950; Kahn & Giffen, 1960; Klopfer et al., 1954; Korchin, 1960; Korchin & Larson, 1977; Lezak, 1976; Mabry, 1964; Neiger et al., 1962; Oberholzer cited in Kisker, 1944; Philippus, 1969; Piotrowski, 1937b; Reitan, 1955c; Rosenzweig & Kogan, 1949; Ross & Ross, 1944; Small, 1973; Weiner, 1966).

13. **Personalized justifications used** (Piotrowski, 1937b; Small, 1973).

14. **Reporting what "the blot is not . . . "** (Evans & Marmorston, 1963, 1964; Weiner, 1977).

15. **An inability to see the popular human figures or seeing a "bird's head" where most people see an *Hd* on Card III** (Ames et al., 1954, 1973; Goldfried et al., 1971).

16. **Rejecting or failing two to five plates** (Philippus, 1969).

Projective Drawing Signs
Graphological and General Indices

1. **Very heavy pressure used** (Buck, 1964; Burgemeister, 1962; DeCato & Wicks, 1976; DiLeo, 1970; Guertin, 1954b; Hammer, 1954c, 1958, 1978; Jacks, 1969; Jolles, 1971; Kahn & Giffen, 1960; Machover, 1949; Michal-Smith, 1953; Payne, 1948; Pope & Scott, 1967; Urban, 1963).

2. **Extreme asymmetry in drawings** (Chase, 1941; Koppitz, 1966c, 1968; Lezak, 1976; Machover, 1949; McElhaney, 1969; Michal-Smith & Morgenstern, 1969; Mundy, 1972; Reynolds, 1978; Rosenzweig & Kogan, 1949; Urban, 1963).

3. **Gross distortions manifested** (Chase, 1941; McElhaney, 1969; Small, 1973; Wiener, 1966).

4. **Very large drawings made** (Kahn & Giffen, 1960; Machover, 1949; Michal-Smith & Morgenstern, 1969; Riklan, Zahn, & Diller, 1962; Urban, 1963).

5. **Erasing with no improvement following the erasing** (Buck, 1948, 1964; Deabler, 1969; Hammer, 1969a, 1978; Jolles, 1971).

6. **Short, discontinuous, or tremulous strokes used** (Adler, 1970; Small, 1973).

7. **Edge of paper prevents completion of the drawing** (DiLeo, 1973).

8. **Perseveration, simplification, or impotency expressions** (Hammer, 1978; Wiener, 1966).

9. **Excessive time is used** (Hammer, 1978).

10. **Omission of one or more essential details** (Hammer, 1978).

Draw-A-Person/Human Figure Drawing Indices

1. **Grossly disorganized or fragmented figures drawn** (Kahn & Giffen, 1960; Koppitz, 1960, 1968; McElhaney, 1969; Modell, 1951; Reznikoff & Tomblen, 1956; Schildkrout et al., 1972; Small, 1973; Weiner, 1966).

2. **Weakly synthesized figures with poor integration** (Kahn & Giffen, 1960; Koppitz, 1968; McElhaney, 1969; Reznikoff & Tomblen, 1956).

3. **Stick figure drawn** (Jacks, 1969; Jolles, 1971).

4. **Lack of detail manifested** (Gilbert, 1969; Kahn & Giffen, 1960).

5. **Unusually large head drawn** (Burgemeister, 1962; Hammer, 1954c, 1978; Jolles, 1971; Kahn & Giffen, 1960; Levy, 1950, 1958; Machover, 1949, 1951; Urban, 1963).

6. **Head drawn with an irregular contour** (Machover, 1949, 1951; McElhaney, 1969; Schildkrout et al., 1972).

7. **Head drawn out of alignment or "floating in space"** (Burgemeister, 1962; Jordan, 1970).

8. **Head omitted from drawing** (DiLeo, 1970; Lezak, 1976).

9. **Confusion of profile and full face in drawing** (Evans & Marmorston, 1963; Machover, 1949; Reznikoff & Tomblen, 1956; Urban, 1963; Zimmerman & Garfinkle, 1942).

10. **Facial features omitted** (Evans & Marmorston, 1963; Lezak, 1976; Schildkrout et al., 1972).

11. **Neck omitted from drawing** (Koppitz, 1968; Lezak, 1976; Mundy, 1972; Schildkrout et al., 1972).

12. **Trunk omitted from drawing** (Gurvitz, 1951; Kahn & Giffen, 1960; Lezak, 1976; Machover, 1949; McElhaney, 1969; Mundy, 1972; Urban, 1963).

13. **Shoulders omitted from drawing** (Burton & Sjoberg, 1964; Evans & Marmorston, 1963; Holzberg & Wexler, 1950; Lezak, 1976).

14. **Dehumanized figures, boxy, robot-, geometric-, manikin-, or monster-like drawings** (Bruell & Albee, 1962; Burgemeister, 1962; Hammer, 1954c; Small, 1973).

15. **Frail, flimsy, thin, wasted, shrunken arms drawn** (Brown, 1953; Buck, 1964, 1966; Hammer, 1954c, 1958; Jolles, 1971; Machover, 1949; Mursell, 1969; Reznikoff & Tomblen, 1956; Urban, 1963; Wolk, 1969).

16. **Hands omitted from the drawing** (Buck, 1948, 1964, 1966; DiLeo, 1973; Evans & Marmorston, 1963; Gilbert, 1969; Halpern, 1958; Hammer, 1953a, 1958, 1960; Koppitz, 1966b, 1966c, 1968; Lezak, 1976; Mundy, 1972; Mursell, 1969; Schildkrout et al., 1972; Urban, 1963).

17. **Petal or grape-like fingers drawn** (Reznikoff & Tomblen, 1956; Schildkrout et al., 1972; Wolk, 1969).

18. **Scribbled fingers** (Reznikoff & Tomblen, 1956).

19. **Thin, tiny, shaded, wasted shrunken legs drawn with a full body** (Hammer, 1958; Machover, 1949; Reznikoff & Tomblen, 1956; Urban, 1963).

20. **Feet omitted from drawing** (Buck, 1948, 1950, 1966; Evans & Marmorston, 1963; Hammer, 1954c; Jolles, 1971; Lezak, 1976; Schildkrout et al., 1972; Urban, 1963).

21. **Stance drawn slanting with legs floating off into space** (Deabler, 1969; Lezak, 1976; Machover, 1949).

22. **Less than two articles of clothing drawn** (Evans & Marmorston, 1963; Koppitz, 1968).

23. **Transparent clothing drawn** (Schildkrout et al., 1972).

24. **Figure drawing developmental level or quotient significantly less than the Stanford-Binet or Wechsler level of intellectual functioning** (Hammer, 1978).

H-T-P House Drawing Indices

1. **Inability to integrate the parts of a House drawing into a unified whole, especially when accompanied by wavy, uneven line quality or poorly connected lines** (Burgemeister, 1962; Hammer, 1969a; Jacks, 1969).

2. **Difficulty in drawing angles on the House** (Deabler, 1969).

3. **Blueprint or a floor plan drawn for a House** (Hammer, 1954c; Jacks, 1969; Jolles, 1971).

4. **An anthropomorphic house drawn** (Jolles, 1971; Zimmerman & Garfinkle, 1942).

5. **Double perspective to House drawing with narrow end walls or with both end walls exaggerated** (Jolles, 1971).

6. **Disconnected or transparent walls drawn** (Jolles, 1971).

7. **Chimney drawn on an angle** (Buck, 1964; Jolles, 1971).

8. **Steps drawn leading to a blank wall** (Jolles, 1971).

9. **House drawing is significantly poorer than the person drawing** (Hammer, 1978).

10. **House is drawn in front view with no side walls shown, or box-like with a blueprint effect** (Hammer, 1978).

11. **Labeling of house parts or rooms** (Hammer, 1978).

H-T-P Tree Drawing Indices

1. **Split Tree drawing with two one-dimensional trees side by side, each with an independent branch structure though also drawn by schizophrenics** (Buck, 1948; Deabler, 1969; Hammer, 1954c, 1958, 1978; Jolles, 1971; Koch, 1952; Landisberg, 1958; Levine & Sapolsky, 1969).

2. **One-dimensional branches drawn inadequately related to one another and inadequately joined to the trunk as in fragmentation or "segmentalization"** (Buck, 1948, 1964; Hammer, 1954c, 1978; Jolles, 1971).

3. **One-dimensional trunks drawn with unorganized one-dimensional branches** (Buck, 1964, 1966; Hammer, 1978; Jolles, 1958, 1971).

4. **Transparent roots or trunks seen through the groundline** (Jolles, 1971).

5. **The Person drawing appears inferior to the Tree drawing** (Jacks, 1969).

6. **The House drawing appears inferior to the Tree drawing** (Deabler, 1969; Hammer, 1954c).

7. **Trees drawn so as to resemble bugs or centipedes** (Hammer, 1978).

Bender-Gestalt Signs
Unusual Reproductive Modes and Arrangements

1. **Angulation changes** (Bender, 1938; Burgemeister, 1962; DeCato & Wicks, 1976; DiLeo, 1970, 1973; Evans & Marmorston, 1963; Hain, 1964; Halpern, 1951; Hutt, 1953, 1977, 1978; Hutt & Briskin, 1960; Hutt & Gibby, 1970; Kahn & Giffen, 1960; Koppitz, 1962; Mosher & Smith, 1965; Quast, 1961; Schneider & Spivack, 1979; Shapiro et al., 1957; Weiner, 1966; Wiener, 1966).

2. **Concreteness, giving Bender figures specific interpretive meanings** (Hain, 1964; Halpern, 1951; Kahn & Giffen, 1960; Lezak, 1976).

3. **Covering a part of the Bender figures when reproducing another part** (Small, 1973).

4. **Curvature modified significantly, especially if angles are introduced** (DeCato & Wicks, 1976; Guertin, 1954b; Halpern, 1951; Koppitz, 1962, 1964; Quast, 1961; Wiener, 1966).

5. **Displacement, parts of the figure related in a bizarre way** (Halpern, 1951; Small, 1973).

6. **Dots changed to circles** (Clawson, 1962; Small, 1973).

7. **Dots changed to dashes** (Mosher & Smith, 1965; Small, 1973).

8. **Dots changed to lines** (Koppitz, 1964; Small, 1973).

9. **Dots changed to loops** (Lerner, 1972; Small, 1973; Tolor, 1968).

10. **Expansion in size of reproductions** (Clawson, 1959; Goldberg, 1956-57; Guertin, 1954a, Kahn & Giffen, 1960; Quast, 1961; Schneider & Spivack, 1979; Woltmann, 1950).

11. **Fragmentation manifested** (Allen, 1958; Bender, 1938; Burgemeister, 1962; Clawson, 1962; Evans & Marmorston, 1963; Feldman, 1953; Gilbert, 1969; Halpern, 1951; Hutt, 1953, 1968, 1977, 1978; Hutt & Gibby, 1970; Kahn & Giffen, 1960; Koppitz, 1962, 1964; Lezak, 1976; Mark & Morrow, 1955; Pascal & Suttell, 1951; Quast, 1961; Schneider & Spivack, 1979).

12. **Expressions of impotence on the Bender, the recognition of an unsatisfactory response and an inability to improve on it** (Small, 1973).

13. **An inability to maintain a horizontal line** (Guertin, 1954b; Mosher & Smith, 1965).

14. **Overlapping and crossing difficulty** (Baroff, 1957; DiLeo, 1973; Evans & Marmorston, 1963; Feldman, 1953; Gilbert, 1969; Hain, 1964; Halpern, 1951; Hutt, 1953, 1977, 1978; Hutt & Briskin, 1960; Hutt & Gibby, 1970; Kahn & Giffen, 1960; Lerner, 1972; Mosher & Smith, 1965; Pope & Scott, 1967; Weiner, 1966; Wiener, 1966).

15. **Perseverations manifested** (Baroff, 1957; Bender, 1938; Bensberg, 1952; Burgemeister, 1962; Clawson, 1962; DeCato & Wicks, 1976; DiLeo, 1970, 1973; Feldman, 1953; Gilbert, 1969; Hain, 1964; Hutt, 1953, 1977, 1978; Hutt & Gibby, 1970; Kahn & Giffen, 1960; Koppitz, 1958, 1962, 1964; Lerner, 1972; Lezak, 1967; Mark & Morrow, 1955; Mosher & Smith, 1965; Pope & Scott, 1967; Quast, 1961; Sattler, 1974; Small, 1973; Tolor, 1968; Weiner, 1966; Wiener, 1966; Woltmann, 1950).

16. **Reduction in size of reproductions** (Allen, 1958; Bender, 1938; Guertin, 1954b; Hutt, 1953; Kahn & Giffen, 1960; Kaldegg, 1956; Lezak, 1976; Schneider & Spivack, 1979; Woltmann, 1950).

17. **Regression, including simplification, primitivation, and condensation** (Bender, 1938; Bensberg, 1952; Clawson, 1962; Evans & Marmorston, 1963; Halpern, 1951; Hutt, 1953, 1977, 1978; Hutt & Gibby, 1970; Kahn & Giffen, 1960; Koppitz, 1962; Lerner, 1972; Lezak, 1976; Pope & Scott, 1967; Quast, 1961; Tolor, 1968; Tolor & Schulberg, 1963; Woltmann, 1950).

18. **Reversals manifested** (Bensberg, 1952; Burgemeister, 1962; Hain, 1964; Halpern, 1951; Quast, 1961; Yates, 1956).

19. **Rotations manifested** (Allison, 1978; Bender, 1938; Burgemeister, 1962; Chorost, Spivack, & Levine, 1959; Clawson, 1962; DeCato & Wicks, 1976; DiLeo, 1973; Evans & Marmorston, 1963; Fabian, 1945; Gobetz, 1953; Griffith & Taylor, 1960, 1961; Guertin, 1952; Hain, 1964; Halpern, 1951; Halpin, 1955; Hanvik, 1953; Hanvik & Andersen, 1950; Hutt, 1953, 1977, 1978; Hutt & Briskin, 1960; Hutt & Gibby, 1970; Kahn & Giffen, 1960; Kaldegg, 1956; Koppitz, 1962, 1964; Lerner, 1972; Lezak, 1976; Mark & Morrow, 1955; Mundy, 1972; Palmer, 1970; Pope & Scott, 1967; Quast, 1961; Schneider & Spivack, 1979; Small, 1973; Symmes & Rapaport, 1972; Tolor, 1968; Tolor & Schulberg, 1963; Weiner, 1966; Wiener, 1966).

20. **Sequentially increasing distortions** (DeCato & Wicks, 1976).

21. **Shaky, sketchy line quality** (Bender, 1938; Hutt, 1953; Kahn & Giffen, 1960).

22. **Spontaneous elaborations, embellishments, and doodling** (Bender, 1938; Hain, 1964; Hutt, 1977; Hutt & Gibby, 1970; Quast, 1961).

23. **Tremors and incoordination noted** (Clawson, 1962; Hutt, 1953, 1977, 1978; Mosher & Smith, 1965; Pascal & Suttell, 1951).

24. **Turning cards or paper** (Hutt & Gibby, 1970; Small, 1973).

25. **Collision arrangements manifested** (Beck, 1959; Burgemeister, 1962; Clawson, 1962; DeCato & Wicks, 1976; Hain, 1964; Halpern, 1951; Hutt, 1953, 1977, 1978; Hutt & Briskin, 1960; Hutt & Gibby, 1970; Mosher & Smith, 1965; Small, 1973).

26. **Confused or chaotic arrangement noted** (Halpern, 1951; Hutt & Briskin, 1960).

27. **Crowded, compressed, cohesive arrangements** (Bender, 1938; Gilbert, 1969; Goldberg, 1956-57; Guertin, 1955; Halpern, 1951; Hutt, 1968).

28. **Total figure is redrawn** (Hutt, 1977).

Unusual Treatment of Specific Figures

1. **Treating the two parts of Figure A as if they were independent units rather than parts of one gestalt** (Halpern, 1951; Koppitz, 1962).

2. **Inability to copy the diamond in Figure A** (Pope & Scott, 1967).

3. **Inappropriate angulation on Figure A** (Halpern, 1951; Koppitz, 1958, 1962; Shapiro et al., 1957).

4. **Dashes for dots on Figure 1** (Bender, 1938; Burgemeister, 1962; Halpern, 1951).

5. **Straight lines to portray dots on Figure 1** (Bender, 1938; Burgemeister, 1962; Halpern, 1951).

6. **Numerals or letters substituted for dots on Figure 1** (Bender, 1938).

7. **Perseveration on Figure 1 and Figure 2** (Bender, 1938; Feldman, 1953; Goldberg, 1956-57; Halpern, 1951; Koppitz, 1962; Weissman & Roth, 1965).

8. **General difficulty with Figure 1** (Hutt, 1977; Hutt & Briskin, 1960).

9. **Letters or numbers used instead of dots on Figure 1** (Bender, 1938).

10. **Inability to maintain the horizontal shape of Figure 1** (Guertin, 1954b).

11. **Abbreviation of Figure 1** (Hain, 1964).

12. **Perseveration and number distortion on Figure 2** (Baroff, 1957; Feldman, 1953; Guertin, 1954a; Halpern, 1951; Koppitz, 1962; Lerner, 1972).

13. **Rotations or omissions on Figure 2** (Koppitz, 1962).

14. **Any significant difficulty in reproducing Figure 2** (Hutt & Briskin, 1960), **especially dots substituted for circles** (Hutt, 1977).

15. **Irregular slope or shifting or abbreviation of Figure 2** (Guertin, 1954a; Hain, 1964; Pope & Scott, 1967).

16. **Dashes for dots on Figure 3** (Bender, 1938; Burgemeister, 1962; Halpern, 1951).

17. **Inappropriate angulation on Figure 3** (Halpern, 1951).

18. **"A flock of birds" seen as a concrete reproduction of Figure 3** (Halpern, 1951).

19. **Fragmentation on Figure 4** (Hutt & Briskin, 1960).

20. **Inappropriate angulation on Figure 4** (Halpern, 1951; Shapiro et al., 1957).

21. **Closure of open figure on Figure 4** (Pope & Scott, 1967).

22. **Lines substituted for dots on Figure 5** (Burgemeister, 1962; Halpern, 1951; Koppitz, 1962; Pope & Scott, 1967).

23. **Dashes or circles substituted for dots on Figure 5** (Burgemeister, 1962; Halpern, 1951).

24. **Squaring of the hoop on Figure 5** (Bender, 1938).

25. **Asymmetry of contour on Figure 6** (Guertin, 1954b).

26. **Nonintersection of lines on Figure 6** (Feldman, 1953; Hutt, 1977).

27. **Straight lines or angles drawn for curves on Figure 6** (Mark & Morrow, 1955).

28. **Total separation of hexagons on Figure 7, or the two tips barely touching** (Feldman, 1953; Hutt & Briskin, 1960; Koppitz, 1958, 1962).

29. **Poor or inappropriate angulation on Figure 7** (Halpern, 1951).

30. **Treating the parts of Figure 7 as if they were independent units rather than as parts of one gestalt** (Halpern, 1951; Hutt, 1977).

31. **Angulation distortions on Figure 8** (Halpern, 1951; Koppitz, 1962).

LOCALIZED AND FOCALIZED BRAIN DAMAGE

Test Indices of Right (or Nondominant) Hemisphere Damage

Wechsler, Bender-Gestalt, and Projective Drawing Signs

1. **VIQ significantly greater than PIQ** (Allen, 1947, 1948a, 1948b; Allison, 1978; Allison et al., 1968; Andersen, 1951; Balthazar et al., 1961; Beck & Lam, 1955; Blatt & Allison, 1968; Boll, 1978; Bruell & Albee, 1962; Davis et al., 1971; Dennerll, 1964; DiLeo, 1973; Fields & Whitmyre, 1969; Fisher, 1960; K.B. Fitzhugh & L.C. Fitzhugh, 1964; Fitzhugh et al., 1962; Goldfarb, 1961; Guertin et al., 1966; Heilbrun, 1956; Hirt & Cook, 1962; Karlin et al., 1959; Kaspar & Schul-

man, 1972; Kaufman, 1979; Klove, 1959, 1974; Klove & Fitzhugh, 1962; Klove & Reitan, 1958; Kohn & Dennis, 1974; Ladd, 1964; Maloney & Ward, 1976; Meier, 1974; Morrow & Mark, 1955; Pope & Scott, 1967; Rabin & McKinney, 1972; Reed & Reitan, 1963; Reitan, 1955c, 1974; Russell, 1979; Russell et al., 1970; Satz, 1966; Satz, Richard, & Daniels, 1967; Simpson & Vega, 1971; Sinnett & Mayman, 1960; Small, 1973; Smith, 1962, 1974; Wechsler, 1958; Zimmerman et al., 1970; Zimmerman & Woo-Sam, 1973) **or this may reflect nondominant hemisphere damage** (Lezak, 1976).

2. **Unusually low Block Design score** (Aita, Armitage, Reitan, & Rabinowitz, 1947; Allison et al., 1968; Balthazar, 1963; Balthazar et al., 1961; Bendien, 1957; Burgemeister, 1962; Davis et al., 1971; Fitzhugh et al., 1962; Glasser & Zimmerman, 1967; Golden, 1976; Gonen, 1970; Greenblatt et al., 1946; Guertin et al., 1966; Heilbrun, 1956, 1959; Hirt & Cook, 1962; Lezak, 1976; Morrow & Mark, 1955; Parker, 1957; Parsons et al., 1963; Rappaport, 1953; Reitan, 1955c, 1964; Russell, 1979; Russell et al., 1970; Small, 1973; Smith, 1966, 1969; Wechsler, 1958; Zimmerman et al., 1970).

3. **Unusually low Digit Symbol score** (Aita, Armitage, Reitan, & Rabinowitz, 1947; Allen, 1947, 1948a, 1948b; Balthazar, 1963; K.B. Fitzhugh & L.C. Fitzhugh, 1964; Gonen, 1970; Guertin et al., 1966; Hirt & Cook, 1962; Hopkins, 1964; Jordan, 1970; Kaspar & Schulman, 1972; Ladd, 1964; Levine & Feirstein, 1972; Magaret, 1942; Morrow & Mark, 1955; Reitan, 1955c, 1974; Reitan & Reed, 1962; Russell, 1972, 1979; Simpson & Vega, 1971; Small, 1973; Smith, 1966, 1974; Stevens et al., 1967; Wechsler, 1958; Zimmerman et al., 1970).

4. **Unusually low Object Assembly score** (Allen, 1947, 1948a; Golden, 1976; Guertin et al., 1966; Kaufman, 1979; Lezak, 1976; Russell, 1979; Russell et al., 1970; Schafer, 1948; Simpson & Vega, 1971; Smith, 1966, 1974; Wechsler, 1958; Zimmerman et al., 1970) **or this may reflect nondominant hemisphere damage** (Lezak, 1976).

5. **Failure on Wechsler block counting yet passing hard Arithmetic items** (Lezak, 1976).

6. **Unusually low Picture Arrangement score, or this may reflect nondominant hemisphere damage** (Heilbrun, 1956; Lezak, 1976; Russell, 1979; Smith, 1969).

7. **Vocabulary score significantly greater than the Block Design score** (Meier, 1974; Parsons, Vega, & Burn, 1969).

8. **Unusually low Digits Backward** (Kaufman, 1979).

9. **Rotation of Bender figures** (Billingslea, 1963; Lezak, 1976).

10. **Drawings done energetically with many strokes** (McFie & Zangwill, 1960).

Rorschach Signs

1. **Unusually low *F%*** (Hall, Hall, & Lavoie, 1968).

2. **Unusually high number of *F-* responses** (Hall et al., 1968).

3. **Unusually high number of responses** (Hall et al., 1968).

4. **Unusually high number of *M*** (Hall et al., 1968).

5. **Unusually high number of shading responses** (Hall et al., 1968).

6. **Fabulized responses present** (Hall et al., 1968).

Test Indices of Left (or Dominant) Hemisphere Damage

Wechsler and Projective Drawing Signs

1. **PIQ is significantly greater than VIQ** (Andersen, 1951; Balthazar, 1963; Balthazar & Morrison, 1961; Balthazar et al., 1961; Boll, 1978; Fields & Whitmyre, 1969; K.B. Fitzhugh & L.C. Fitzhugh, 1964; Fitzhugh et al., 1962; Guertin et al., 1966; Heilbrun, 1956; Klove, 1959, 1974; Klove & Reitan, 1958; Maloney & Ward, 1976; Meyer & Jones, 1957; Reitan, 1955c, 1974; Russell, 1979; Russell et al., 1970; Satz, 1966; Satz et al., 1967; Simpson & Vega, 1971; Smith, 1962; Zimmerman & Woo-Sam, 1973).

2. **Unusually low Digit Span score** (Heilbrun, 1956; Lezak, 1976; McFie, 1960; Russell, 1972; Russell et al., 1970; Small, 1973; Smith, 1974; Zimmerman & Woo-Sam, 1973) **especially low Digits Forward** (Kaufman, 1979).

3. **Unusually low Information score** (Fitzhugh et al., 1962; Smith, 1966), **or this may reflect dominant hemisphere damage** (Lezak, 1976).

4. **Unusually low Similarities score** (Heilbrun, 1956; Kaufman, 1979; Lezak, 1976; McFie, 1960; Reitan, 1964; Russell et al., 1970; Small, 1973; Smith, 1966).

5. **Unusually low Comprehension score** (Fitzhugh et al., 1962; Heilbrun, 1956; Smith, 1966), **or this may reflect dominant hemisphere damage** (Lezak, 1976).

6. **Vocabulary score significantly less than Block Design score** (Kaufman, 1979; Parsons et al., 1969; Russell et al., 1970).

7. **Unusually low Arithmetic score** (Russell et al., 1970).

Table 1
Points to be Added for Age-Scaled Scores

Age Group	Vocabulary	Similarities	Arithmetic	Digit Span	Picture Completion	Picture Arrangement	Block Designs	Digit Symbol
30–34	0	0	1	1	1	1	0	1
35–39	0	0	1	1	1	1	1	1
40–44	0	1	1	1	1	2	1	2
45–49	0	1	1	1	2	2	2	2
50–54	0	1	1	2	2	3	2	3
55–59	0	2	2	2	2	3	3	3
60–64	1	2	2	3	3	4	3	4
65–69	1	3	3	3	3	5	4	5

Note. Reprinted by permission from McFie (1975).

8. **A very long drawing time** (McFie & Zangwill, 1960).

Rorschach Signs

1. **An unusually small number of responses** (Hall et al., 1968).
2. **Perplexity expressed** (Hall et al., 1968).
3. **Rejections or failures manifested** (Hall et al., 1968).
4. **An unusually high *F%*** (Hall et al., 1968).

IMPAIRMENT FROM FOCALIZED BRAIN DAMAGE

McFie (1975) articulated a technique primarily utilizing Wechsler data (and some other test data not embraced by this volume) to generate interpretive hypotheses regarding the site of focal brain damage. Concern regarding not using an extensive test battery is attenuated by a pair of studies. In one, Watson et al. (1968) presented data which suggested that predictions made on the basis of the full Halstead-Reitan battery were no better than those from the WAIS alone. Another study by Lacks et al. (1970) concluded that the Bender-Gestalt predicted organicity as well as or better than the Halstead tests. They also confirmed the finding of Watson et al. that the Halstead battery is of little help for differential diagnoses between organics and non-organic psychotics. In the meantime, appropriate though cautious interpretive hypotheses regarding the site of central nervous system damage may be generated from the battery of tests reported in this section.

McFie suggested that Wechsler subtest patterns should display age-corrected scaled scores. He derived these age-scaled scores for pertinent subtests from the work of Wechsler (1944) and Fox and Birren (1950). For those who wish to use them, the correction values are presented in Table 1. Of course, distinct profiles frequently are not appreciably altered by these corrections.

Test Indices

Wechsler and Bender-Gestalt Signs

The following test sign interpretive hypothesis relationships may be tendered, though they may be considered most appropriate for the 90% of the population who are right-handed.

1. *Left frontal area adversely affected* **is suggested by high Picture Completion, Vocabulary, and Block Design scores with low Digit Span and Digit Symbol scores** (McFie, 1975).
2. *Left temporal lobe affected adversely* **is suggested by high Picture Completion and Block Design scores with low Similarities, Digit Span, and Digit Symbol scores** (Kunce et al., 1976; Lezak, 1976; McFie, 1975; Meyer & Jones, 1957), **and sometimes low Vocabulary** (McFie, 1960; Milberg et al., 1980), **and the VIQ significantly below the PIQ** (Meyer & Jones, 1957).
3. *Left parietal area affected adversely* **is suggested by high Vocabulary and Picture Completion scores with low Arithmetic, Digit Symbol, Digit Span, and Block Design scores** (McFie, 1975).
4. *Right frontal area affected adversely* **is suggested by high Picture Completion, Vocabulary, Similarities, and Arithmetic scores with low Digit Symbol and Picture Arrangement scores** (McFie, 1975) **or a tendency to leave the Picture Arrangement pictures in the order presented** (McFie & Thompson, 1972).

5. *Right temporal area affected adversely* is suggested by high Picture Completion, Similarities, Arithmetic, Vocabulary, and Digit Span scores with low Digit Symbol and Picture Arrangement scores (Hutt, 1977; Lezak, 1976; McFie, 1975; Meier, 1974; Meier & French, 1965; Reitan, 1955b, 1974); **the low Picture Arrangement scores have been associated with damage to the right anterior temporal lobe** (Lezak, 1976; Meier, 1974; Meier & French, 1965; Reitan, 1955b, 1974).

6. *Right parietal area affected adversely* is suggested by high Similarities, Vocabulary, and Picture Completion scores with low Block Design, Digit Symbol, and Picture Arrangement scores (Kaufman, 1979; Lezak, 1976; McFie, 1975; Reitan, 1974), **or Bender rotations** (Hirschenfang, 1970; Lezak, 1976).

Contraindications

Wechsler Signs

1. **Block Design scaled score unusually high** (Gurvitz, 1951; Patterson, 1953; Wechsler, 1958).

Rorschach Signs

1. *FM* **greater than** *2M* (Goldfried et al., 1971; Hughes, 1948, 1950).
2. *M + m* **greater than 2** (Dorken & Kral, 1952; Goldfried et al., 1971).

3. **Better than average quality** *F* **responses** (Gottlieb & Parsons, 1960).
4. *FK + K + k* **greater than zero** (Dorken & Kral, 1952; Goldfried et al., 1971).
5. *Fc + FC* **greater than 2** (Dorken & Kral, 1952; Goldfried et al., 1971).
6. *S* **responses emphasized** (Dorken & Kral, 1952).
7. *O* **responses present in greater than average number and with satisfactory form levels** (Dorken & Kral, 1952; Goldfried et al., 1971).
8. **Confused (less than three systematic) sequences** (Goldfried et al., 1971; Hughes, 1948, 1950).
9. **An unusually large number of responses** (Dorken & Kral, 1952; Goldfried et al., 1971).
10. **Color shock to Card II** (Goldfried et al., 1971; Hughes, 1948, 1950).
11. **Shading shock to Card V** (Goldfried et al., 1971; Hughes, 1948, 1950).

Projective Drawing and Bender-Gestalt Signs

1. **Frequent erasures manifested with subsequent improvement in the drawing** (Ogdon, 1975).
2. **Correct reproduction of Bender-Gestalt Figure 7** (Weissman & Roth, 1965).
3. **Projective drawings are well organized and effectively executed** (Hammer, 1978).
4. **Split Tree and anthropomorphic House drawings are not drawn by organics (though these have been associated with schizophrenia)** (Hammer, 1978).

CHAPTER 7
PROGNOSES

The dimension of prognoses ranges from very good to very poor. Surveying the psychological literature on the subject (Ogdon, 1975) led to the conclusion that prognostications based on test data, beyond the admittedly artificial dichotomy of Favorable and Unfavorable, may not be warranted at this time. The expression of a guarded prognosis appears to be a guarded expression of an unfavorable prediction.

Most psychological test indices relevant to prognosticating appear on Rorschach's test, and most of those are associated with Klopfer's (1954) *Rorschach Prognostic Rating Scale* (e.g., Davids & Talmadge, 1964; Goldfried et al., 1971; Klopfer et al., 1954). Garwood's work (1977, 1978), as well as the work of Newmark, Finkelstein, and Frerking (1974) and Newmark, Hetzel, Walker, Holstein, and Finkelstein (1973), is largely supportive of the efficacy of the *Rorschach Prognostic Rating Scale* for a variety of types of patients treated with various therapeutic techniques. Windle (1952) and Hiler (1958) have pertinent findings to present regarding prognostic signs on the Wechsler, and Hammer (1953c, 1969a) has presented comparable observations of projective drawing indices. Beyond these signs, one may deduce that indices of chronic brain damage or of psychosis, especially schizophrenia, suggest a poorer prognosis than signs of neuroses or of borderline conditions. Within limits, younger patients tend to have more favorable prognoses than elderly ones.

Behavioral manifestations which may be associated with clinical prognoses, other than response to therapy and spontaneous remissions, do not appear to have received sufficient study to justify further consideration of them in this volume.

Test Indices of Favorable Prognoses

Wechsler Signs

1. **Similarities score unusually high** (Hiler, 1958; Windle, 1952).
2. **Picture Completion score unusually high** (Windle, 1952).
3. **Block Design score unusually high** (Windle, 1952).
4. **Picture Arrangement score unusually high** (Windle, 1952).
5. **Object Assembly score unusually high** (Windle, 1952).

Rorschach Signs

1. *M* **responses present in greater than average number** (Allen, 1954, 1958; Dana, 1968; Davids & Talmadge, 1964; Garwood, 1977, 1978; Goldfried et al., 1971; King, 1958, 1960; Klopfer & Davidson, 1962; Newmark et al., 1973, 1974; Nickerson, 1969; Phillips & Smith, 1953; Piotrowski, 1937a, 1957, 1960, 1969, 1977; Piotrowski & Bricklin, 1961; Schumer cited in Sarason, 1954; Singer, 1955, 1960; Weiner, 1977).
2. *M+* **responses present** (Exner, 1974; Garwood, 1977, 1978; Goldfried et al., 1971; Klopfer et al., 1954; Newmark et al., 1973, 1974; Weiner, 1977).
3. *FM* **present in an unusually large number** (Garwood, 1977, 1978; Goldfried et al., 1971; Klopfer et al., 1954; Newmark et al., 1973, 1974; Weiner, 1977).
4. *FM+* **responses present** (Klopfer et al., 1954).
5. *M + m* **significantly greater than 2, especially if inanimate movement is countergravity and form dominated** (Garwood, 1977, 1978; Goldfried et al., 1971; Klopfer et al., 1954; Newmark et al., 1973, 1974; Weiner, 1977).
6. *FC* **present in greater than average number** (Garwood, 1977, 1978; Goldfried et al., 1971; Klopfer et al., 1954; Newmark et al., 1973, 1974; Weiner, 1977).
7. *Fc* **present in greater than average number, especially with "warm" or "soft" responses** (Garwood, 1977, 1978; Goldfried et al., 1971; Klopfer et al., 1954; Newmark et al., 1973, 1974; Weiner, 1977).
8. **Vista** *(FK)* **responses present in greater than average number** (Garwood, 1977, 1978; Goldfried et al., 1971; Klopfer et al., 1954; Newmark et al., 1973, 1974; Weiner, 1977).
9. *H* **content present in greater than average number** (Garwood, 1977, 1978; Goldfried et al., 1971; Klopfer et al., 1954; Newmark et al., 1973, 1974; Weiner, 1977).
10. *R* **greater than average** (Weiner, 1977).
11. **Better than average overall form level** (Garwood, 1977, 1978; Goldfried et al., 1971; Klopfer et al., 1954; Newmark et al., 1973, 1974; Weiner, 1977).

Projective Drawing Signs

1. **The Tree drawing appears healthier than the Person drawing** (Hammer, 1953c, 1969a).

2. **Satisfactory drawing of facial features** (Fiedler & Siegel, 1949).

Test Indices of Unfavorable Prognoses

Rorschach Signs

1. **Subnormal quality of *F* responses** (Allen, 1954; Beck, 1944, 1945, 1951, 1968; Berkowitz & Levine, 1953; Bohm, 1958; Garwood, 1977, 1978; Goldfried et al., 1971; Gottlieb & Parsons, 1960; Hertz & Paolino, 1960; Holt, 1968; Kahn & Giffen, 1960; Kalinowsky & Hoch, 1961; Kataguchi, 1959; Klopfer et al., 1954; Korchin, 1960; Neiger et al., 1962; Newmark et al., 1973, 1974; Phillips & Smith, 1953; Piotrowski, 1957; Piotrowski & Berg, 1955; Piotrowski & Bricklin, 1961; Piotrowski & Lewis, 1950; Rapaport et al., 1946; Schafer, 1948, 1954, 1960; Weiner, 1961b, 1977; Wolman, 1972).

2. **Subnormal number of *M* responses** (Affleck & Mednick, 1959; Davids & Talmadge, 1964; Garwood, 1977, 1978; Goldfried et al., 1971; Kaden & Lipton, 1960; Klopfer et al., 1954; Newmark et al., 1973, 1974; Piotrowski, 1960, 1969; Piotrowski & Bricklin, 1961; Weiner, 1977).

3. ***M-* responses present** (Garwood, 1977, 1978; Goldfried et al., 1971; Klopfer et al., 1954; Newmark et al., 1973, 1974; Weiner, 1977).

4. **Subnormal number of *FM* responses** (Garwood, 1977, 1978; Goldfried et al., 1971; Klopfer et al., 1954; Newmark et al., 1973, 1974; Weiner, 1977).

5. ***FM-* responses present** (Garwood, 1977, 1978; Goldfried et al., 1971; Klopfer et al., 1954; Newmark et al., 1973, 1974; Weiner, 1977).

6. ***Fm-* responses present** (Garwood, 1977, 1978; Goldfried et al., 1971; Klopfer et al., 1954; Newmark et al., 1973, 1974; Weiner, 1977).

7. **Flexor *M* responses given in significant number** (Beck, 1945).

8. **Sum *C* greater than *2M*, particularly when *M*: Sum *C* is beyond 1:3 and *M* is 0 or 1** (Piotrowski & Bricklin, 1961; Rapaport et al., 1946; Schafer, 1948, 1954; Vinson, 1960).

9. ***F%* is greater than 50** (Adams et al., 1963; Davids & Talmadge, 1964; Mundy, 1972).

10. ***FC + CF + C* approximately zero** (Adams et al., 1963; Arnaud, 1959; Davids & Talmadge, 1964; Harrower-Erickson, 1941; Levine et al., 1957; Sarason, 1954; Schachtel, 1943; Wagner, 1971).

11. **Sum *C* greater than *M* + 3 when *M* is 0 or 1** (Piotrowski, 1969).

12. ***FC-* responses given** (Garwood, 1977, 1978; Goldfried et al., 1971; Klopfer et al., 1954; Newmark et al., 1973, 1974; Weiner, 1977).

13. ***CF-* responses given** (Garwood, 1977, 1978; Goldfried et al., 1971; Klopfer et al., 1954; Newmark et al., 1973, 1974; Weiner, 1977).

14. **Pure *C* responses present** (Garwood, 1977, 1978; Goldfried et al., 1971; Klopfer et al., 1954; Newmark et al., 1973, 1974; Weiner, 1977).

15. ***Cn* responses present** (Garwood, 1977, 1978; Goldfried et al., 1971; Klopfer et al., 1954; Newmark et al., 1973, 1974; Weiner, 1977).

16. **Poor quality *Fc* responses present** (Garwood, 1977, 1978; Goldfried et al., 1971; Klopfer et al., 1954; Newmark et al., 1973, 1974; Weiner, 1977).

17. **Pure *c* responses present** (Garwood, 1977, 1978; Goldfried et al., 1971; Klopfer et al., 1954; Newmark et al., 1973, 1974; Weiner, 1977).

18. **Poor quality Vista *(FK)* responses present** (Garwood, 1977, 1978; Goldfried et al., 1971; Klopfer et al., 1954; Newmark et al., 1973, 1974; Weiner, 1977).

19. **Animal responses given in greater than normal number** (Davids & Talmadge, 1964).

20. ***H + Hd* responses equal to zero** (Piotrowski, 1969).

21. **Few content categories utilized** (Allison et al., 1968; Evans & Marmorston, 1963; Olch, 1971; Piotrowski & Bricklin, 1961; Sherman, 1955).

22. **Failures or rejections manifested** (Carnes & Bates, 1971; Davids & Talmadge, 1964).

23. **Perplexity expressed** (Piotrowski, 1969; Vinson, 1960).

Projective Drawing Signs

1. **Facial features omitted from a human figure drawing** (Fiedler & Siegel, 1949).
2. **Tree drawing is a dead tree** (Hammer, 1958).
3. **The drawn Person appears healthier than the Tree drawing** (Hammer, 1953c, 1969a).

REFERENCES

Acker, C.W. Personality concomitants of autonomic balance I: Rorschach measures. *Journal of Projective Techniques*, 1963, *27*, 12–19.

Adams, H., Cooper, G., & Carrera, R. The Rorschach and the MMPI: A concurrent validity study. *Journal of Projective Techniques*, 1963, *27*, 23–34.

Adler, P.T. Evaluation of the figure drawing technique: Reliability, factorial structure, and diagnostic usefulness. *Journal of Consulting and Clinical Psychology*, 1970, *35*, 52–57.

Affleck, D.C., & Mednick, S.A. The use of the Rorschach test in the prediction of the abrupt terminator in individual psychotherapy. *Journal of Consulting Psychology*, 1959, *23*, 125–128.

Aita, J.A., Armitage, S.G., Reitan, R.M., & Rabinowitz, A. The use of certain psychological tests in the evaluation of brain injury. *Journal of General Psychology*, 1947, *37*, 25–44.

Aita, J.A., Reitan, R.M., & Ruth, J.M. Rorschach's test as a diagnostic aid in brain injury. *American Journal of Psychiatry*, 1947, *103*, 770–779.

Alcock, T. *The Rorschach in practice*. Philadelphia: Lippincott, 1963.

Alexander, F. *Fundamentals of psychoanalysis*. New York: Norton, 1948.

Alexander, F., Crutchlow, E., & Hoffman, M. A selective survey of the Wechsler-Bellevue section of Rapaport's *Diagnostic psychological testing. Canadian Journal of Psychology*, 1947, *1*, 111–115.

Allen, R.M. The test performance of the brain injured. *Journal of Clinical Psychology*, 1947, *3*, 225–230.

Allen, R.M. A note on the use of the Bellevue-Wechsler scale mental deterioration index with brain injured patients. *Journal of Clinical Psychology*, 1948, *4*, 88–89. (a)

Allen, R.M. II. The test performance of the brain diseased. *Journal of Clinical Psychology*, 1948, *4*, 281–284. (b)

Allen, R.M. *Elements of Rorschach interpretation*. New York: International Universities Press, 1954.

Allen, R.M. *Personality assessment procedures*. New York: Harper & Row, 1958.

Allison, J. Clinical contributions of the Wechsler Adult Intelligence Scale. In B.B. Wolman (Ed.), *Clinical diagnosis of mental disorders: A handbook*. New York: Plenum Publishing Corp., 1978.

Allison, J., Blatt, S.J., & Zimet, C.N. *The interpretation of psychological tests*. New York: Harper & Row, 1968.

Allport, G. *Personality: A psychological interpretation*. New York: Holt, 1937.

Alschuler, A., & Hattwick, W. *Painting and personality*. Chicago: University of Chicago Press, 1947.

Altus, W.D., & Clark, J.H. Subtest variation on the Wechsler-Bellevue for two institutionalized behavior problem groups. *Journal of Consulting Psychology*, 1949, *13*, 444–447.

American Psychiatric Association. *Diagnostic and statistical manual of mental disorders* (3rd ed.). Washington, D.C.: Author, 1980.

Ames, L.B., & Gillespie, C. Significance of Rorschach response modified by responses to other projective tests. *Journal of Personality Assessment*, 1973, *37*, 316–327.

Ames, L.B., Learned, J., Metraux, R., & Walker, R.N. *Child Rorschach responses*. New York: Hoeber, 1952.

Ames, L.B., Learned, J., Metraux, R., & Walker, R.N. *Rorschach responses in old age*. New York: Hoeber, 1954.

Ames, L.B., Metraux, R., Rodell, J., & Walker, R.N. *Rorschach responses in old age* (2nd ed.). New York: Brunner/ Mazel, 1973.

Ames, L.B., Metraux, R.W., Rodell, J.L., & Walker, R.N. *Child Rorschach responses* (Rev. ed.). New York: Brunner/ Mazel, 1974.

Ames, L.B., Metraux, R., & Walker, R.N. *Adolescent Rorschach responses*. New York: Hoeber, 1959.

Ames, L.B., Metraux, R., & Walker, R.N. *Adolescent Rorschach responses* (2nd ed.). New York: Brunner/ Mazel, 1971.

Andersen, A.L. The effect of laterality localization of focal brain lesions on the Wechsler-Bellevue subtests. *Journal of Clinical Psychology*, 1951, *7*, 149–153.

Andersen, D.O., & Seitz, F.C. Rorschach diagnosis of homosexuality: Schafer's content analysis. *Journal of Projective Techniques and Personality Assessment*, 1969, *33*, 406–408.

Anthony, W.Z., Heaton, R.K., & Lehman, R.A.W. An attempt to cross-validate two actuarial systems for neuropsychological test interpretation. *Journal of Consulting and Clinical Psychology*, 1980, *48*, 317–326.

Appelbaum, S., & Colson, D. A reexamination of the color-shading Rorschach test response and suicide attempts. *Journal of Projective Techniques and Personality Assessment*, 1968, *32*, 160–164.

Appelbaum, S., & Holzman, P.S. The color-shading response and suicide. *Journal of Projective Techniques*, 1962, *26*, 155–161.

Armon, V. Some personality variables in overt female homosexuality. *Journal of Projective Techniques*, 1960, *24*, 292–309.

Arnaud, S. A system for deriving quantitative Rorschach measures of certain psychological variables, for group comparisons. *Journal of Projective Techniques*, 1959, *23*, 403–411.

Aronoff, J. Sex differences in the orientation of body image. *Journal of Personality Assessment*, 1972, *36*, 19–22.

Aronow, E., & Reznikoff, M. *Rorschach content interpretation*. New York: Grune & Stratton, 1976.

Aronson, M.L. A study of the Freudian theory of paranoia by means of the Rorschach test. *Journal of Projective Techniques*, 1952, *16*, 397–411.

Auerbach, S.M., & Spielberger, C.D. The assessment of state and trait anxiety. *Journal of Personality Assessment*, 1972, *36*, 314–335.

Baker, G. Diagnosis of organic brain damage in the adult. In B. Klopfer (Ed.), *Developments in the Rorschach technique. Vol. II. Fields of application*. New York: Harcourt Brace Jovanovich, 1956.

Baker, L.M., & Harris, J. The validation of Rorschach test results against laboratory behavior. *Journal of Clinical Psychology*, 1949, *5*, 161–164.

Baldwin, I.T. The head-body ratio in human figure drawings of schizophrenic and normal adults. *Journal of Projective Techniques and Personality Assessment*, 1964, *28*, 393–396.

Balthazar, E.E. Cerebral unilateralization in chronic epileptic cases: The Wechsler Object Assembly subtest. *Journal of Clinical Psychology*, 1963, *19*, 169–171.

Balthazar, E.E., & Morrison, D.H. The use of Wechsler intelligence scales as diagnostic indicators of predominant left-right and indeterminate unilateral brain damage. *Journal of Clinical Psychology*, 1961, *17*, 161–165.

Balthazar, E.E., Todd, R.E., Morrison, D.H., & Ziebell, P.W. Visuoconstructive and verbal responses in chronic brain-damaged patients and familial retardates. *Journal of Clinical Psychology*, 1961, *17*, 293–296.

Barnouw, V. Cross-cultural research with the House-Tree-Person test. In J.N. Buck & E.F. Hammer (Eds.), *Advances in the House-Tree-Person technique: Variations and applications*. Los Angeles: Western Psychological Services, 1969.

Baroff, G.S. Bender-Gestalt visuo-motor function in mental deficiency. *American Journal of Mental Deficiency*, 1957, *61*, 753–760.

Barrell, R.P. Subcategories of Rorschach human movement responses: A classification system and some experimental results. *Journal of Consulting Psychology*, 1953, *17*, 254–260.

Barron, F. Threshold for the perception of human movement in inkblots. *Journal of Consulting Psychology*, 1955, *19*, 33–38.

Beck, H.S. A study of the applicability of the H-T-P to children with respect to the drawn house. *Journal of Clinical Psychology*, 1955, *11*, 60–63.

Beck, H.S. A comparison of convulsive organics, non-convulsive organics, and non-organic public school children. *American Journal of Mental Deficiency*, 1959, *63*, 866–875.

Beck, H.S., & Lam, R.L. Use of the WISC in predicting organicity. *Journal of Clinical Psychology*, 1955, *11*, 154–158.

Beck, S.J. *Rorschach's test. I. Basic processes*. New York: Grune & Stratton, 1944.

Beck, S.J. *Rorschach's test. II. A variety of personality pictures*. New York: Grune & Stratton, 1945.

Beck, S.J. The Rorschach test: A multi-dimensional test of personality. In H.H. Anderson & G. Anderson (Eds.), *An introduction to projective techniques*. Englewood Cliffs, N.J.: Prentice-Hall, 1951.

Beck, S.J. *Rorschach's test. III. Advances in interpretation*. New York: Grune & Stratton, 1952.

Beck, S.J. *The Rorschach experiment*. New York: Grune & Stratton, 1960.

Beck, S.J. Reality, Rorschach and perceptual theory. In A.I. Rabin (Ed.), *Projective techniques in personality assessment*. New York: Springer Publishing Co., Inc., 1968.

Beck, S.J. *Rorschach test: Vol. 2. Gradients in mental disorder* (3rd ed.). New York: Grune & Stratton, 1978.

Beck, S.J., Beck, A.G., Levitt, E.E., & Molish, H.B. *Rorschach's test. I. Basic processes* (3rd ed.). New York: Grune & Stratton, 1961.

Beck, S.J., & Molish, H.B. *Rorschach's test. II. A variety of personality pictures* (2nd ed.). New York: Grune & Stratton, 1967.

Bell, J.E. *Projective techniques*. New York: Longmans, Green, 1948.

Bellak, L. The concept of acting out: Theoretical considerations. In L.E. Abt & S.L. Weissman (Eds.), *Acting out*. New York: Grune & Stratton, 1965.

Bellak, L., & Fielding, C. Diagnosing schizophrenia. In B.B. Wolman (Ed.), *Clinical diagnosis of mental disorders: A handbook*. New York: Plenum Publishing Corp., 1978.

Bender, L. *A Visual Motor Gestalt Test and its clinical use*. New York: American Orthopsychiatric Association, 1938.

Bender, L. *Psychopathology of children with organic brain disorders*. Springfield, IL.: Charles C. Thomas, 1956.

Bendick, M., & Klopfer, W.G. The effects of sensory deprivation and motor inhibition on Rorschach movement responses. *Journal of Projective Techniques*, 1964, *28*, 261–264.

Bendien, J. [A validation study of the Rail-Walking Test.] *Nederlands Tijdschrift voor de Psychologie*, 1957, *12*, 424–455 (Psychological Abstracts, 33:3815).

Bensberg, G. Performance of brain-injured and familial mental defectives on the Bender-Gestalt Test. *Journal of Consulting Psychology*, 1952, *16*, 61–64.

Benton, A.L. Psychological test for brain damage. In A.M. Freedman & H.I. Kaplan (Eds.), *Comprehensive textbook of psychiatry*. Baltimore: Williams & Wilkins, 1967.

Benton, A.L., & Howell, I.L. The use of psychological tests in the evaluation of intellectual function following head injury: Report of a case of post-traumatic personality disorder. *Psychosomatic Medicine*, 1941, *3*, 138–151.

Berkowitz, M., & Levine, J. Rorschach scoring categories as diagnostic "signs." *Journal of Consulting Psychology*, 1953, *17*, 110–112.

Bernstein, R., & Corsini, R.J. Wechsler-Bellevue patterns of female delinquents. *Journal of Clinical Psychology*, 1953, *9*, 176–179.

Billingslea, F.Y. The Bender-Gestalt: An objective scoring method and validating data. *Journal of Clinical Psychology*, 1948, *4*, 1–27.

Billingslea, F.Y. The Bender-Gestalt: A review and perspective. *Psychological Bulletin*, 1963, *60*, 233–251.

Birch, H.G., & Diller, L. Rorschach signs of "organicity": A physiological basis for perceptual disturbances. *Journal of Projective Techniques*, 1959, *23*, 184–197.

Black, F.W. Cognitive deficits in patients with unilateral war-related frontal lobe lesions. *Journal of Clinical Psychology*, 1976, *32*, 366–376.

Blank, L. The intellectual functioning of delinquents. *Journal of Social Psychology*, 1958, *47*, 9–14.

Blatt, S.J. The Wechsler scales and acting out. In L. Abt & S. Weissman (Eds.), *Acting out*. New York: Grune & Stratton, 1965.

Blatt, S.J., & Allison, J. The intelligence test in personality assessment. In A.I. Rabin (Ed.), *Projective techniques in personality assessment*. New York: Springer Publishing Co., Inc., 1968.

Blatt, S.J., Allison, J., & Baker, B.L. The Wechsler Object Assembly subtest and bodily concerns. *Journal of Consulting Psychology*, 1965, *29*, 223–230.

Blatt, S.J., Brenneis, C.B., Shimek, J.G., & Glick, M. Normal development and psychopathological impairment on the concept of the object on the Rorschach. *Journal of Abnormal Psychology*, 1976, *85*, 364–373.

Blatt, S.J., & Quinlan, P. Punctual and procrastinating students: A study of temporal parameters. *Journal of Consulting Psychology*, 1967, *31*, 169–174.

Blatt, S.J., & Ritzler, B.A. Suicide and the representation of transparency and cross-sections on the Rorschach. *Journal of Consulting and Clinical Psychology*, 1974, *42*, 280–287.

Bloom, B.L. The Rorschach popular response among Hawaiian schizophrenics. *Journal of Projective Techniques*, 1962, *26*, 173–181.

Bochner, R., & Halpern, F. *The clinical application of the Rorschach test*. New York: Grune & Stratton, 1945.

Bodwin, R.F., & Bruck, M. The adaptation and validation of the Draw-A-Person test as a measure of self concept. *Journal of Clinical Psychology*, 1960, *16*, 427–429.

Bohm, E. *A textbook in Rorschach test diagnosis*. New York: Grune & Stratton, 1958.

Bohm, E. The Binder chiaroscuro system and its theoretical basis (M. Felix, trans.). In M. Rickers-Ovsiankina (Ed.), *Rorschach psychology*. New York: John Wiley & Sons, Inc., 1960.

Bohm, E. The Binder chiaroscuro system and its theoretical basis. In M. Rickers-Ovsiankina (Ed.), *Rorschach psychology* (2nd ed.). New York: Krieger, 1977.

Boll, T.J. Diagnosing brain impairment. In B.B. Wolman (Ed.), *Clinical diagnosis of mental disorders: A handbook*. New York: Plenum Publishing Corp., 1978.

Bradfield, R.H. The predictive validity of children's drawings. *California Journal of Educational Research*, 1964, *15*, 166–174.

Bradway, K., & Benson, S. The application of the method of extreme deviations to Rapaport's Wechsler-Bellevue data. *Journal of Clinical Psychology*, 1955, *11*, 285–291.

Bradway, K., & Heisler, V. The relation between diagnoses and certain types of extreme deviations and content on the Rorschach. *Journal of Projective Techniques*, 1953, *17*, 70–74.

Brannigan, G.G., & Benowitz, M.L. Bender-Gestalt signs and antisocial acting out tendencies in adolescents. *Psychology in the Schools*, 1975, *12*, 15–17.

Brar, H.S. Rorschach content responses of East Indian psychiatric patients. *Journal of Projective Techniques and Personality Assessment*, 1970, *34*, 88–94.

Brick, M. Mental hygiene value of children's art work. *American Journal of Orthopsychiatry*, 1944, *14*, 136–146.

Broida, D.C. An investigation of certain psychodiagnostic indications of suicidal tendencies and depression in mental hospital patients. *Psychiatric Quarterly*, 1954, *28*, 453–464.

Brown, F. An exploratory study of dynamic factors in the content of the Rorschach protocol. *Journal of Projective Techniques*, 1953, *17*, 251–279.

Brown, F. Adult case study: Clinical validation of the House-Tree-Person drawings of an adult case (chronic ulcerative colitis with ileostomy). In E.F. Hammer (Ed.), *The clinical application of projective drawings*. Springfield, IL.: Charles C. Thomas, 1958.

Brown, F. The Bender-Gestalt and acting out. In L. Abt & S. Weissman (Eds.), *Acting out*. New York: Grune & Stratton, 1965.

Brown, F., Chase, J., & Winson, J. Studies in infant feeding choices of primiparae. *Journal of Projective Techniques*, 1961, *25*, 412–421.

Bruell, J.H., & Albee, G.W. Higher intellectual functions in a patient with hemispherectomy for tumors. *Journal of Consulting Psychology*, 1962, *26*, 90–98.

Bruhn, A.R., & Reed, M.R. Simulation of brain damage on the Bender-Gestalt test by college students. *Journal of Personality Assessment*, 1975, *39*, 244–255.

Buck, J.N. The H-T-P technique, a qualitative and quantitative scoring manual. *Journal of Clinical Psychology*, 1948, *4*, 317–396.

Buck, J.N. The use of the House-Tree-Person test in a case of marital discord. *Journal of Projective Techniques*, 1950, *14*, 405–434.

Buck, J.N. *The House-Tree-Person (H-T-P) manual supplement, administration and interpretation of the H-T-P test*. Los Angeles: Western Psychological Services, 1964.

Buck, J.N. *The House-Tree-Person technique: Revised manual*. Los Angeles: Western Psychological Services, 1966.

Buck, J.N. The use of the H-T-P in the investigation of the dynamics of intra-familial conflict. In J.N. Buck & E.F. Hammer (Eds.), *Advances in the House-Tree-Person technique: Variations and applications*. Los Angeles: Western Psychological Services, 1969.

Burgemeister, B.B. *Psychological techniques in neurological diagnosis*. New York: Hoeber-Harper, 1962.

Burton, A., & Sjoberg, B. The diagnostic validity of human figure drawings in schizophrenia. *Journal of Psychology*, 1964, *57*, 3–18.

Byrd, E. The clinical validity of the Bender Gestalt Test with children: A developmental comparison of children in need of psychotherapy and children judged well-adjusted. *Journal of Projective Techniques*, 1956, *20*, 127–136.

Carlson, K., Quinlan, D., Tucker, G., & Harrow, M. Body disturbance and sexual elaboration factors in figure drawings of schizophrenic patients. *Journal of Personality Assessment*, 1973, *37*, 56–63.

Carnes, G.D., & Bates, R. Rorschach anatomy response correlates in rehabilitation failure subjects. *Journal of Personality Assessment*, 1971, *35*, 527–537.

Cerbus, G., & Nichols, R.C. Personality variables and response to color. *Psychological Bulletin*, 1963, *60*, 566–575.

Chase, J.M. A study of the drawings of a male figure made by schizophrenic patients and normal subjects. *Character & Personality*, 1941, *9*, 208–217.

Chorost, S., Spivack, G., & Levine, M. Bender-Gestalt rotations and EEG abnormalities in children. *Journal of Consulting Psychology*, 1959, *23*, 559.

Clark, J.H. Intelligence test results obtained from a specific type of army A.W.O.L. *Educational and Psychological Measurement*, 1948, *8*, 677–682.

Clawson, A. The Bender Visual Motor Gestalt Test as an index of emotional disturbance in children. *Journal of Projective Techniques*, 1959, *23*, 198–206.

Clawson, A. *The Bender Visual Motor Gestalt Test for children: A manual*. Los Angeles: Western Psychological Services, 1962.

Coates, S. Homosexuality and the Rorschach test. *British Journal of Medical Psychology*, 1962, *35*, 177–190.

Cocking, R.R., Dana, J.M., & Dana, R.H. Six constructs to define Rorschach M: A response. *Journal of Projective Techniques and Personality Assessment*, 1969, *33*, 322–323.

Coleman, J.C. *Abnormal psychology and modern life*. Glenview, IL.: Scott, Foresman & Co., 1972.

Coleman, J.C., & Rasof, B. Intellectual factors in learning disorders. *Perceptual & Motor Skills*, 1963, *16*, 139–152.

Colson, D.B., & Hurwitz, B.A. A new experimental approach to the relationship between color-shading and suicide attempts. *Journal of Personality Assessment*, 1973, *37*, 237–241.

Consalvi, C., & Canter, A. Rorschach scores as a function of four factors. *Journal of Consulting Psychology*, 1957, *21*, 47–51.

Cooper, L. Motility and fantasy in hospitalized patients. *Perceptual and Motor Skills*, 1969, *28*, 525–526.

Cooper, L., & Caston, J. Physical activity and increase in M response. *Journal of Projective Techniques and Personality Assessment*, 1970, *34*, 295–301.

Costello, C.G. The Rorschach records of suicidal patients. *Journal of Projective Techniques*, 1958, *22*, 272–275.

Cox, F.N., & Sarason, S.B. Test anxiety and Rorschach performance. *Journal of Abnormal and Social Psychology*, 1954, *49*, 371–377.

Crenshaw, D.A., Bohn, S., Hoffman, M., Matheus, J.M., & Offenbach, S.G. The use of projective methods in research: 1947–1965. *Journal of Projective Techniques and Personality Assessment*, 1968, *32*, 3–9.

Curnutt, R.H. The use of the Bender-Gestalt with an alcoholic and non-alcoholic population. *Journal of Clinical Psychology*, 1953, *9*, 287–290.

Cutter, F., Jorgenson, M., & Farberow, N.L. Replicability of Rorschach signs with known degrees of suicidal intent. *Journal of Projective Techniques and Personality Assessment*, 1968, *32*, 428–434.

Dana, R.H. Six constructs to define Rorschach M. *Journal of Projective Techniques and Personality Assessment*, 1968, *32*, 138–145.

Dana, R.H., & Cocking, R.R. Cue parameters, cue probabilities, and clinical judgment. *Journal of Clinical Psychology*, 1968, *24*, 475–480.

Daston, P.G., & Sakheim, G.A. Prediction of successful suicide from the Rorschach test, using a sign approach. *Journal of Projective Techniques*, 1960, *24*, 355–361.

Davids, A., Joelson, M., & McArthur, C. Rorschach and TAT indices of homosexuality in overt homosexuals, neurotics, and normal males. *Journal of Abnormal and Social Psychology*, 1956, *53*, 161–172.

Davids, A., & Talmadge, M. Utility of the Rorschach in predicting movement in psychiatric care work. *Journal of Consulting Psychology*, 1964, *28*, 311–316.

Davidson, H. A measure of adjustment obtained from the Rorschach protocol. *Journal of Projective Techniques*, 1950, *14*, 31–38.

Davis, W.E., Becker, B.C., & DeWolfe, A.S. Categorization of patients with personality disorders and acute brain trauma through WAIS subtest variations. *Journal of Clinical Psychology*, 1971, *27*, 358–360.

Davis, W.E., DeWolfe, A.S., & Gustafson, R.C. Intellectual deficit in process and reactive schizophrenia and brain injury. *Journal of Consulting and Clinical Psychology*, 1972, *38*, 146.

Davison, L.A. Current status of clinical neurology. In R.M. Reitan & L.A. Davison (Eds.), *Clinical neuropsychology: Current status and applications*. New York: Halstead Press, 1974.

Deabler, H.L. The H-T-P in group testing and as a screening device. In J.N. Buck & E.F. Hammer (Eds.), *Advances in the House-Tree-Person technique: Variations and applications*. Los Angeles: Western Psychological Services, 1969.

DeCato, C.M., & Wicks, R.J. *Case studies of the clinical interpretation of the Bender-Gestalt test*. Springfield, IL.: Charles C. Thomas, 1976.

DeCourcy, P. The hazard of short-term psychotherapy without assessment: A case history. *Journal of Personality Assessment*, 1971, *35*, 285–288.

DeKoninck, J.M., & Crabbe-Decleve, G. Field dependence and Rorschach white-space figure-ground reversal responses. *Perceptual and Motor Skills*, 1971, *33*, 1191–1194.

DeLuca, J.N. The structure of homosexuality. *Journal of Projective Techniques and Personality Assessment*, 1966, *30*, 187–191.

DeMartino, M.F. Human figure drawings by mentally retarded males. *Journal of Clinical Psychology*, 1954, *10*, 241–244.

Dennerll, R.D. Prediction of unilateral brain dysfunction using Wechsler test scores. *Journal of Consulting Psychology*, 1964, *28*, 278–284.

Dennerll, R.D., Broeder, J., & Sokolov, S.L. WISC and WAIS factors in children and adults with epilepsy. *Journal of Clinical Psychology*, 1964, *20*, 236–237.

DeVos, G. A quantitative approach to affective symbolism in Rorschach responses. *Journal of Projective Techniques*, 1952, *16*, 133–150.

DeWolfe, A.S. Differentiation of schizophrenia and brain damage with the WAIS. *Journal of Clinical Psychology*, 1971, *27*, 209–211.

DeWolfe, A.S., Barrell, R.P., Becker, B.C., & Spaner, F.E. Intellectual deficit in chronic schizophrenia and brain damage. *Journal of Consulting Psychology*, 1971, *36*, 197–204.

DiLeo, J.H. *Young children and their drawings*. New York: Brunner/Mazel, 1970.

DiLeo, J.H. *Children's drawings as diagnostic aids*. New York: Brunner/Mazel, 1973.

Diller, L. A comparison of the test performances of delinquent and non-delinquent girls. *Journal of Genetic Psychology*, 1952, *81*, 167–183.

Doris, J., Sarason, S.B., & Berkowitz, L. Test anxiety and performance on projective tests. *Child Development*, 1963, *34*, 751–766.

Dorken, H., & Kral, V.A. The psychological differentiation of organic brain lesions and their localization by means of the Rorschach test. *American Journal of Psychiatry*, 1952, *108*, 764–770.

DuBrin, A.J. The Rorschach "eyes" hypothesis and paranoid schizophrenia. *Journal of Clinical Psychology*, 1962, *18*, 468–471.

Dudek, S.Z. Intelligence, psychopathology and primary thinking disorders in early schizophrenia. *Journal of Nervous and Mental Disease*, 1969, *148*, 515–527.

Dudek, S.Z. A longitudinal study of Piaget's developmental stages and the concept of regression. II. *Journal of Personality Assessment*, 1972, *36*, 468–478.

Due, F.O., & Wright, M.E. The use of content analysis in Rorschach interpretation: I. Differential characteristics of male homosexuals. *Rorschach Research Exchange*, 1945, *9*, 169–177.

Eichler, R.M. Experimental stress and alleged Rorschach indices of anxiety. *Journal of Abnormal and Social Psychology*, 1951, *46*, 344–355.

Eisenthal, S. Assessment of suicide risk using selected tests. In C. Neuringer (Ed.), *Psychological assessment of suicidal risk*. Springfield, IL.: Charles C. Thomas, 1974.

Elizur, A. Content analysis of the Rorschach with regard to anxiety and hostility. *Journal of Projective Techniques*, 1949, *13*, 247–284.

Elstein, A.S. Behavioral correlates of the Rorschach shading determinant. *Journal of Consulting Psychology*, 1965, *29*, 231–236.

Endicott, N.A., & Jortner, S. Objective measures of depression. *Archives of General Psychiatry*, 1966, *15*, 249–255.

Endicott, N.A., Jortner, S., & Abramoff, E. Objective measures of suspiciousness. *Journal of Abnormal Psychology*, 1969, *74*, 26–32.

English, H.B., & English, A.C. *A comprehensive dictionary of psychological and psychoanalytical terms*. New York: Longmans, Green, 1958.

Erickson, R.C., Calsyn, D.A., & Scheupbach, C.S. Abbreviating the Halstead-Reitan neuropsychological test battery. *Journal of Clinical Psychology*, 1978, *34*, 922–926.

Evans, R.B., & Marmorston, J. Psychological test signs of brain damage in cerebral thrombosis. *Psychological Reports*, 1963, *12*, 915–930.

Evans, R.B., & Marmorston, J. Rorschach signs of brain damage in cerebral thrombosis. *Perceptual and Motor Skills*, 1964, *18*, 977–988.

Exner, J.E. A comparison of the human figure drawings of psychoneurotics, character disturbances, normals, and subjects experiencing experimentally-induced fear. *Journal of Projective Techniques*, 1962, *26*, 392–397.

Exner, J.E., Jr. Rorschach responses as an index of narcissism. *Journal of Projective Techniques and Personality Assessment*, 1969, *33*, 324–330. (a)

Exner, J.E., Jr. *The Rorschach systems*. New York: Grune & Stratton, 1969. (b)

Exner, J.E., Jr. *The Rorschach: A comprehensive system*. New York: John Wiley & Sons, Inc., 1974.

Exner, J.E., Jr. *The Rorschach: A comprehensive system. Vol. 2: Current research and advanced interpretation*. New York: John Wiley & Sons, Inc., 1978.

Exner, J.E., & Clark, B. The Rorschach. In B.B. Wolman (Ed.), *Clinical diagnosis of mental disorders: A handbook*. New York: Plenum Publishing Corp., 1978.

Exner, J.E., Jr., & Wylie, J. Some Rorschach data concerning suicide. *Journal of Personality Assessment*, 1977, *41*, 339–348.

Fabian, A.A. Vertical rotation in visual-motor performance: Its relationship to reading reversals. *Journal of Educational Psychology*, 1945, *36*, 129–154.

Fein, L.G. Current status of psychological diagnostic testing in university training programs and in delivery of service systems. *Psychological Reports*, 1979, *44*, 863–879.

Feldman, I. Psychological differences among moron and borderline mental defectives as a function of etiology: I. Visual-motor functioning. *American Journal of Mental Retardation*, 1953, *57*, 484–494.

Fenichel, O. *The psychoanalytic theory of neurosis*. New York: Norton, 1945.

Ferguson, L.W. *Personality measurement*. New York: McGraw-Hill, 1952.

Fiedler, F.E., & Siegel, S.M. The Free Drawing Test as a predictor of non-improvement in psychotherapy. *Journal of Clinical Psychology*, 1949, *5*, 386–389.

Fields, F.R.J., & Whitmyre, J.W. Verbal and performance relationships with respect to laterality of cerebral involvement. *Diseases of the Nervous System*, 1969, *30*, 177–179.

Fine, L.G. Rorschach signs of homosexuality in male college students. *Journal of Clinical Psychology*, 1950, *6*, 248–253.

Finney, B. Rorschach test correlates of assaultive behavior. *Journal of Projective Techniques*, 1955, *19*, 6–16.

Fisher, G.C. Selective and differentially accelerated intellectual dysfunction in specific brain damage. *Journal of Clinical Psychology*, 1958, *14*, 395–398.

Fisher, G.M. Differences in WAIS Verbal and Performance IQ's in various diagnostic groups of mental retardates. *American Journal of Mental Deficiency*, 1960, *65*, 256–260.

Fisher, S. Patterns of personality rigidity and some of their determinants. *Psychological Monographs*, 1950, *64* (No. 307).

Fisher, S. Rorschach patterns in conversion hysteria. *Journal of Projective Techniques*, 1951, *15*, 98–108.

Fisher, S. Relationship of Rorschach human percepts to projective descriptions with self reference. *Journal of Projective Techniques*, 1962, *26*, 231–233.

Fisher, S., & Sunukjian, H. Intellectual disparities in a normal group and their relationship to emotional disturbance. *Journal of Clinical Psychology*, 1950, *6*, 288–290.

Fitzhugh, K.B., & Fitzhugh, L.C. WAIS results for Ss with longstanding, chronic, lateralized and diffuse cerebral dysfunction. *Perceptual and Motor Skills*, 1964, *19*, 735–739.

Fitzhugh, K., Fitzhugh, L.C., & Reitan, R.M. Wechsler-Bellevue comparisons in groups with "chronic" and "current" lateralized and diffuse brain lesions. *Journal of Consulting Psychology*, 1962, *26*, 306–310.

Fitzhugh, L.C., & Fitzhugh, K. Relationships between Wechsler-Bellevue Form I and WAIS performances of subjects with longstanding cerebral dysfunction. *Perceptual and Motor Skills*, 1964, *19*, 539–543.

Fonda, C.P. The white-space response. In M. Rickers-Ovsiankina (Ed.), *Rorschach psychology*. New York: John Wiley & Sons, Inc., 1960.

Fonda, C.P. The white-space response. In M. Rickers-Ovsiankina (Ed.), *Rorschach psychology* (2nd ed.). New York: Krieger, 1977.

Foster, A.L. A note concerning the intelligence of delinquents. *Journal of Clinical Psychology*, 1959, *15*, 78–79.

Fox, C., & Birren, J.E. Intellectual deterioration in the aged. *Journal of Consulting Psychology*, 1950, *14*, 305–310.

Franklin, J.C. Discriminative value and patterns of the Wechsler-Bellevue scales in the examination of delinquent Negro boys. *Educational and Psychological Measurement*, 1945, *5*, 71–85.

Freud, S. The sexual aberration. In A.A. Brill (trans.), *The basic writings of Sigmund Freud*. New York: Random House, 1938. (Originally published, 1905).

Freud, S. The psychopathology of everyday life (J. Strachey, Ed., and A. Tyson, trans.). New York: Norton, 1971. (Originally published, 1904).

Friedman, H. Perceptual regression in schizophrenia: An hypothesis suggested by the use of the Rorschach test. *Journal of Genetic Psychology*, 1952, *81*, 63–98.

Friedman, H. Perceptual regression in schizophrenia: An hypothesis suggested by the use of the Rorschach test. *Journal of Projective Techniques*, 1953, *17*, 171–185.

Fukada, N. Japanese children's tree drawings. In J.N. Buck & E.F. Hammer (Eds.), *Advances in the House-Tree-Person technique: Variations and applications*. Los Angeles: Western Psychological Services, 1969.

Fuller, J.B., & Chagnon, G. Factors influencing rotation in the Bender-Gestalt performance of children. *Journal of Projective Techniques*, 1962, *26*, 36–46.

Furrer, A. The meaning of M in the Rorschach test (J. Blauner, trans.). In M. Sherman (Ed.), *A Rorschach reader*. New York: International Universities Press, 1960.

Garfield, S.L. An evaluation of Wechsler-Bellevue patterns in schizophrenia. *Journal of Consulting Psychology*, 1949, *13*, 279–287.

Garwood, J. A guide to research on the Rorschach Prognostic Rating Scale. *Journal of Personality Assessment*, 1977, *41*, 117–119.

Garwood, J. Six-month prognostic norms derived from studies of the Rorschach Prognostic Rating Scale. *Journal of Personality Assessment*, 1978, *42*, 22–26.

Gavales, D., & Millon, T. Comparison of reproduction and recall size deviations in the Bender-Gestalt as measures of anxiety. *Journal of Clinical Psychology*, 1960, *16*, 278–280.

Geil, G.A. The use of the Goodenough test for revealing male homosexuality. *Journal of Criminal Psychopathology*, 1944, *6*, 307–321.

Gilbert, J. *Clinical psychological tests in psychiatric and medical practice*. Springfield, IL.: Charles C. Thomas, 1969.

Glasser, A.J., & Zimmerman, I.L. *Clinical interpretation of the Wechsler Intelligence Scale for Children.* New York: Grune & Stratton, 1967.

Glueck, S., & Glueck, E.T. *Ventures in criminology.* Cambridge, MA.: Harvard University Press, 1964.

Gobetz, W. A quantification, standardization, and validation of the Bender-Gestalt Test on normal and neurotic adults. *Psychological Monographs*, 1953, *67* (No. 356).

Goldberg, F.H. The performance of schizophrenic, retarded, and normal children on the Bender-Gestalt Test. *American Journal of Mental Deficiency*, 1956-57, *61*, 548–555.

Golden, C.J. The identification of brain damage by an abbreviated form of the Halstead-Reitan neuropsychological battery. *Journal of Clinical Psychology*, 1976, *32*, 821–826.

Goldfarb, W. A definition and validation of obsessional trends in the Rorschach examination of adolescents. *Rorschach Research Exchange*, 1943, *7*, 81–108.

Goldfarb, W. *Childhood schizophrenia.* Cambridge, MA.: Harvard University Press, 1961.

Goldfried, M.R. The assessment of anxiety by means of the Rorschach. *Journal of Projective Techniques and Personality Assessment*, 1966, *30*, 364–380. (a)

Goldfried, M.R. On the diagnosis of homosexuality from the Rorschach. *Journal of Consulting Psychology*, 1966, *30*, 338–349. (b)

Goldfried, M.R., Stricker, G., & Weiner, I.B. *Rorschach handbook of clinical and research applications.* Englewood Cliffs, N.J.: Prentice-Hall, 1971.

Goldman, R. Changes in Rorschach performance and clinical improvement in schizophrenia. *Journal of Consulting Psychology*, 1960, *24*, 403–407.

Goldstein, A.P., & Rawn, M.L. The validity of interpretive signs of aggression in the drawing of the human figure. *Journal of Clinical Psychology*, 1957, *13*, 169–171.

Goldstein, H.S., & Faterson, H.F. Shading as an index of anxiety in figure drawings. *Journal of Projective Techniques and Personality Assessment*, 1969, *33*, 454–456.

Gonen, J.Y. The use of Wechsler's deterioration quotient in cases of diffuse and symmetrical cerebral atrophy. *Journal of Clinical Psychology*, 1970, *26*, 174–177.

Goodman, M., & Kotkov, B. Prediction of trait ranks from Draw-A-Person measurements of obese and non-obese women. *Journal of Clinical Psychology*, 1953, *9*, 365–367.

Goodstein, L.D., & Goldberger, L. Manifest anxiety and Rorschach performance in a chronic patient population. *Journal of Consulting Psychology*, 1955, *19*, 339–344.

Gottlieb, A., & Parsons, O. A coaction compass evaluation of Rorschach determinants in brain damaged individuals. *Journal of Consulting Psychology*, 1960, *24*, 54–60.

Graham, E.E., & Kamano, D. Reading failure as a factor in the WAIS subtest patterns of youthful offenders. *Journal of Clinical Psychology*, 1958, *14*, 302–305.

Gray, D.M., & Pepitone, A. Effect of self-esteem on drawings of the human figure. *Journal of Consulting Psychology*, 1964, *28*, 452–455.

Green, R., Fuller, M., & Rutley, B. It-Scale for children and Draw-A-Person Test: 30 feminine vs. 25 masculine boys. *Journal of Personality Assessment*, 1972, *36*, 349–352.

Greenblatt, M., Goldman, R., & Coon, G. Clinical implications of the Wechsler-Bellevue test, with particular reference to cases of injury to the brain. *Archives of Neurology and Psychiatry*, 1946, *56*, 714–717.

Griffith, A.V., & Peyman, D.A.R. Eye-ear emphasis in the DAP as indicating ideas of reference. *Journal of Consulting Psychology*, 1959, *23*, 560.

Griffith, R.M., & Taylor, V.H. Incidence of Bender-Gestalt figure rotations. *Journal of Consulting Psychology*, 1960, *24*, 189–190.

Griffith, R.M., & Taylor, V.H. Bender-Gestalt figure rotations: A stimulus factor. *Journal of Consulting Psychology*, 1961, *25*, 89–90.

Guertin, W. A factor analysis of the Bender-Gestalt tests of mental patients. *Journal of Clinical Psychology*, 1952, *8*, 362–367.

Guertin, W. A factor analysis of curvilinear distortions on the Bender-Gestalt. *Journal of Clinical Psychology*, 1954, *10*, 12–17. (a)

Guertin, W. A transposed analysis of the Bender-Gestalts of brain disease cases. *Journal of Clinical Psychology*, 1954, *10*, 366–369. (b)

Guertin, W. A transposed factor analysis of schizophrenic performance on the Bender-Gestalt. *Journal of Clinical Psychology*, 1954, *10*, 225–228. (c)

Guertin, W. A transposed analysis of the Bender-Gestalts of paranoid schizophrenics. *Journal of Clinical Psychology*, 1955, *11*, 73–76.

Guertin, W., Ladd, C.E., Frank, G.H., Rabin, A.I., & Hiester, D.S. Research with the Wechsler intelligence scales for adults: 1960–1965. *Psychological Bulletin*, 1966, *66*, 385–409.

Gurvitz, M. *The dynamics of psychological testing.* New York: Grune & Stratton, 1951.

Hafner, A.J., & Rosen, E. The meaning of Rorschach inkblots, responses, and determinants as perceived by children. *Journal of Projective Techniques*, 1964, *28*, 192–200.

Hain, J.D. The Bender-Gestalt Test: A scoring method for identifying brain damage. *Journal of Consulting Psychology*, 1964, *28*, 34–40.

Hall, G.S. A synthetic genetic study of fear. *American Journal of Psychology*, 1914, *25*, 149–200.

Hall, M.M., Hall, G.C., & Lavoie, P. Ideation in patients with unilateral or bilateral midline brain lesions. *Journal of Abnormal Psychology*, 1968, *73*, 526–531.

Halpern, F. The Bender Visual Motor Gestalt Test. In H.H. Anderson & G. Anderson (Eds.), *An introduction to projective techniques.* Englewood Cliffs, N.J.: Prentice-Hall, 1951.

Halpern, F. *A clinical approach to children's Rorschachs.* New York: Grune & Stratton, 1953.

Halpern, F. Child case study. In E.F. Hammer (Ed.), *The clinical application of projective drawings.* Springfield, IL.: Charles C. Thomas, 1958.

Halpern, F. The Rorschach test with children. In A.I. Rabin & M.R. Haworth (Eds.), *Projective techniques with children.* New York: Grune & Stratton, 1960.

Halpern, F. Diagnostic methods in childhood disorders. In B.B. Wolman (Ed.), *Handbook of clinical psychology.* New York: McGraw-Hill, 1965.

Halpin, V. Rotation errors made by brain injured and familial children on two visual motor tests. *American Journal of Mental Deficiency,* 1955, *59,* 485–489.

Halstead, W.C. *Brain and intelligence.* Chicago: University of Chicago Press, 1947.

Hammer, E.F. An investigation of sexual symbolism: A study of H-T-P's of eugenically sterilized subjects. *Journal of Projective Techniques,* 1953, *17,* 401–413. (a)

Hammer, E.F. Negro and white children's personality adjustment as revealed by a comparison of their drawings (H-T-P). *Journal of Clinical Psychology,* 1953, *9,* 7–10. (b)

Hammer, E.F. The role of the H-T-P in the prognostic battery. *Journal of Clinical Psychology,* 1953, *9,* 371–374. (c)

Hammer, E.F. A comparison of H-T-P's of rapists and pedophiles. *Journal of Projective Techniques,* 1954, *18,* 346–354. (a)

Hammer, E.F. An experimental study of symbolism on the Bender-Gestalt. *Journal of Projective Techniques,* 1954, *18,* 335–345. (b)

Hammer, E.F. Guide for qualitative research with the H-T-P. *Journal of General Psychology,* 1954, *51,* 41–60. (c)

Hammer, E.F. A comparison of H-T-P's of rapists and pedophiles: III. The "dead" tree as an index of psychopathology. *Journal of Clinical Psychology,* 1955, *11,* 67–69.

Hammer, E.F. *The clinical application of projective drawings.* Springfield, IL.: Charles C. Thomas, 1958.

Hammer, E.F. The House-Tree-Person (H-T-P) drawings as a projective technique with children. In A.I. Rabin & M.R. Haworth (Eds.), *Projective techniques with children.* New York: Grune & Stratton, 1960.

Hammer, E.F. Acting out and its prediction by projective drawing assessment. In L. Abt & S. Weissman (Eds.), *Acting out.* New York: Grune & Stratton, 1965.

Hammer, E.F. Projective drawings. In A.I. Rabin (Ed.), *Projective techniques in personality assessment.* New York: Springer, 1968.

Hammer, E.F. Hierarchal organization of personality and the H-T-P, achromatic and chromatic. In J.N. Buck & E.F. Hammer (Eds.), *Advances in the House-Tree-Person technique: Variations and applications.* Los Angeles: Western Psychological Services, 1969. (a)

Hammer, E.F. The use of the H-T-P in a criminal court: Predicting acting out. In J.N. Buck & E.F. Hammer (Eds.), *Advances in the House-Tree-Person technique: Variations and applications.* Los Angeles: Western Psychological Services, 1969. (b)

Hammer, E.F. Projective drawings: Two areas of differential diagnostic challenge. In B.B. Wolman (Ed.), *Clinical diagnosis of mental disorders: A handbook.* New York: Plenum Publishing Corp., 1978.

Hammes, J.A., & Osborne, R.T. Discrimination of manifest anxiety by the structural-objective Rorschach test. *Perceptual and Motor Skills,* 1962, *15,* 59–62.

Handler, L., & Reyher, J. The effects of stress on the Draw-A-Person Test. *Journal of Consulting Psychology,* 1964, *28,* 259–264.

Handler, L., & Reyher, J. Figure drawing anxiety indices: A review of the literature. *Journal of Projective Techniques,* 1965, *29,* 305–313.

Handler, L, & Reyher, J. Relationship between GSR and anxiety indexes in projective drawings. *Journal of Consulting Psychology,* 1966, *30,* 60–67.

Hanvik, L.J. A note on rotations in the Bender Gestalt Test as predictors of EEG abnormalities in children. *Journal of Clinical Psychology,* 1953, *9,* 399.

Hanvik, L.J., & Andersen, A.L. The effect of focal brain lesions on recall and on the production of rotations in the Bender-Gestalt Test. *Journal of Consulting Psychology,* 1950, *14,* 197–198.

Hardison, J., & Purcell, K. The effects of psychological stress as a function of need and cognitive control. *Journal of Personality,* 1959, *27,* 250–258.

Harris, J.G., Jr. Validity: The search for a constant in a universe of variables. In M. Rickers-Ovsiankina (Ed.), *Rorschach psychology.* New York: John Wiley & Sons, Inc., 1960.

Harris, R. A comparative study of two groups of boys, delinquent and non-delinquent, on the basis of their Wechsler and Rorschach test performance. *Bulletin of the Maritime Psychological Association,* 1957, *6,* 21–28.

Harrow, M., Quinlan, D., Wallington, S., & Pickett, L., Jr. Primitive drive-dominated thinking: Relationship to acute schizophrenia and sociopathy. *Journal of Personality Assessment,* 1976, *40,* 31–41.

Harrower, M. The measurement of psychological factors in marital maladjustment. In V.W. Eisenstein (Ed.), *Neurotic interaction in marriage.* New York: Basic Books, 1956.

Harrower-Erickson, M. Personality changes accompanying organic brain lesions: III. A study of preadolescent children. *Journal of Genetic Psychology,* 1941, *58,* 391–445.

Haskell, R.J., Jr. Relationship between aggressive behavior and psychological tests. *Journal of Projective Techniques,* 1961, *25,* 431–440.

Hassell, J., & Smith, E.W.L. Female homosexuals' concepts of self, men, and women. *Journal of Personality Assessment,* 1975, *39,* 154–159.

Haworth, M. Responses of children to a group projective film and to the Rorschach, CAT, Despert Fables and D-A-P. *Journal of Projective Techniques,* 1962, *26,* 47–60.

Haworth, M., & Rabin, A.I. Miscellaneous techniques. In A.I. Rabin & M. Haworth (Eds.), *Projective techniques with children.* New York: Grune & Stratton, 1960.

Hays, J.R., Solway, K.S., & Schreiner, D. Intellectual characteristics of juvenile murderers versus status offenders. *Psychological Reports*, 1978, *43*, 80–82.

Heaton, R.K., Smith, H.H., Jr., Lehman, R.A.W., & Vogt, A.T. Prospects for faking believable deficits on neuropsychological testing. *Journal of Consulting and Clinical Psychology*, 1978, *46*, 892–900.

Heaton, R.K., Vogt, A.T., Hoehn, M.M., Lewis, J.A., Crowley, T.J., & Stallings, M.A. Neuropsychological impairment with schizophrenia vs. acute and chronic cerebral lesions. *Journal of Clinical Psychology*, 1979, *35*, 46–53.

Heilbrun, A.B., Jr. Psychological test performance as a function of lateral localization of cerebral lesion. *Journal of Comparative and Physiological Psychology*, 1956, *49*, 10–14.

Heilbrun, A.B., Jr. The digit span test and the prediction of cerebral pathology. *Archives of Neurology and Psychiatry*, 1958, *80*, 228–231.

Heilbrun, A.B., Jr. Lateralization of cerebral lesion and performance on spatial-temporal tasks. *Archives of Neurology*, 1959, *1*, 282–287.

Henrichs, T.F., & Amolsch, T.J. A note on the actuarial interpretation of WAIS profile patterns. *Journal of Personality Assessment*, 1978, *42*, 418–420.

Hersch, C. The cognitive functioning of the creative person: A developmental analysis. *Journal of Projective Techniques*, 1962, *26*, 193–200.

Hertz, M. Suicidal configurations in Rorschach records. *Rorschach Research Exchange and Journal of Projective Techniques*, 1948, *12*, 3–58.

Hertz, M. Further study of "suicidal" configurations in Rorschach records. *Rorschach Research Exchange and Journal of Projective Techniques*, 1949, *13*, 44–73.

Hertz, M. The organization activity. In M. Rickers-Ovsiankina (Ed.), *Rorschach psychology*. New York: John Wiley & Sons, Inc., 1960. (a)

Hertz, M. The Rorschach in adolescence. In A.I. Rabin & M. Haworth (Eds.), *Projective techniques with children*. New York: Grune & Stratton, 1960. (b)

Hertz, M. Detection of suicidal risks with the Rorschach. In L. Abt & S. Weissman (Eds.), *Acting out*. New York: Grune & Stratton, 1965.

Hertz, M., & Loehrke, L.M. The application of the Piotrowski and Hughes signs of organic defect to a group of patients suffering from post-traumatic encephalopathy. *Journal of Projective Techniques*, 1954, *18*, 183–196.

Hertz, M., & Paolino, A. Rorschach indices of perceptual and conceptual disorganization. *Journal of Projective Techniques*, 1960, *24*, 370–388.

Hetherington, R. The effects of E.C.T. on the drawings of depressed patients. *Journal of Mental Science*, 1952, *98*, 450–453.

Hewson, L.R. The Wechsler-Bellevue Scale and the substitution test as aids in neuropsychiatric diagnosis. *Journal of Nervous and Mental Disease*, 1949, *109*, 158–183; 264–266.

Hiler, E. Wechsler-Bellevue intelligence as a predictor of continuation in psychotherapy. *Journal of Clinical Psychology*, 1958, *14*, 192–194.

Hinsie, L.E., & Campbell, R.J. *Psychiatric dictionary*. London: Oxford University Press, 1970.

Hirschenfang, S. A comparison of Bender-Gestalt reproductions of right and left hemiplegic patients. *Journal of Clinical Psychology*, 1960, *16*, 439.

Hirt, M.L., & Cook, R.A. Use of a multiple regression equation to estimate organic impairment from Wechsler scale scores. *Journal of Clinical Psychology*, 1962, *18*, 80–81.

Holland, T.R., Levi, M., & Watson, C.G. Multivariate structure of associations between verbal and non-verbal intelligence among brain-damaged, schizophrenic, neurotic, and alcoholic patients. *Journal of Abnormal Psychology*, 1979, *88*, 354–360.

Holland, T.R., & Watson, C.G. Multivariate analysis of WAIS-MMPI relationships among brain-damaged, schizophrenic, neurotic, and alcoholic patients. *Journal of Clinical Psychology*, 1980, *36*, 352–359.

Holt, R.R. *Diagnostic psychological testing* (Rev. ed.). New York: International Universities Press, 1968.

Holzberg, J.D., & Wexler, M. The validity of human form drawings as a measure of personality deviation. *Journal of Projective Techniques*, 1950, *14*, 343–361.

Hooker, E. Male homosexuality in the Rorschach. *Journal of Projective Techniques*, 1958, *22*, 33–54.

Hopkins, K.D. An empirical analysis of the efficacy of the WISC in the diagnosis of organicity in children of normal intelligence. *Journal of Genetic Psychology*, 1964, *105*, 163–172.

Hoyt, T.E., & Baron, M.R. Anxiety indices in same-sex drawings of psychiatric patients with high and low MAS scores. *Journal of Consulting Psychology*, 1959, *23*, 448–452.

Hozier, A. On the breakdown of the sense of reality: A study of spatial perception in schizophrenia. *Journal of Consulting Psychology*, 1959, *23*, 185–194.

Hughes, R.M. Rorschach signs for the diagnosis of organic pathology. *Rorschach Research Exchange*, 1948, *12*, 165–167.

Hughes, R.M. A factor analysis of Rorschach diagnostic signs. *Journal of General Psychology*, 1950, *43*, 85–103.

Hutt, M.L. Revised Bender Visual-Motor Gestalt Test. In A. Weider (Ed.), *Contributions toward medical psychology: Theory and psychodiagnostic methods. Vol. II*. New York: Ronald Press Co., 1953.

Hutt, M.L. The projective use of the Bender-Gestalt Test. In A.I. Rabin (Ed.), *Projective techniques in personality assessment*. New York: Springer Publishing Co., Inc., 1968.

Hutt, M.L. *The Hutt adaptation of the Bender-Gestalt Test* (3rd ed.). New York: Grune & Stratton, 1977.

Hutt, M.L. The Hutt adaptation of the Bender-Gestalt Test: Diagnostic and therapeutic implications. In B.B. Wolman (Ed.), *Clinical diagnosis of mental disorders: A handbook*. New York: Plenum Publishing Corp., 1978.

Hutt, M.L., & Briskin, G.J. *The clinical use of the Revised Bender-Gestalt Test.* New York: Grune & Stratton, 1960.

Hutt, M.L., & Gibby, R.G. *An atlas for the Hutt adaptation of the Bender-Gestalt Test.* New York: Grune & Stratton, 1970.

Ingram, W. Prediction of aggression from the Rorschach. *Journal of Consulting Psychology,* 1954, *18,* 23–28.

Jacks, I. The clinical application of the H-T-P in criminological settings. In J.N. Buck & E. F. Hammer (Eds.), *Advances in the House-Tree-Person technique: Variations and applications.* Los Angeles: Western Psychological Services, 1969.

Jackson, C.V. Estimating impairment on Wechsler Bellevue subtests. *Journal of Clinical Psychology,* 1955, *11,* 137–143.

Johnson, J.H. Upper left hand placement of human figure drawings as an indicator of anxiety. *Journal of Personality Assessment,* 1971, *35,* 336–337.

Johnson, J.H. Bender-Gestalt constriction as an indicator of depression in psychiatric patients. *Journal of Personality Assessment,* 1973, *37,* 53–55.

Jolles, I. A study of the validity of some hypotheses for the qualitative interpretation of the H-T-P for children of elementary school age: I. Sexual identification. *Journal of Clinical Psychology,* 1952, *8,* 113–118. (a)

Jolles, I. A study of the validity of some hypotheses for the qualitative interpretation of the H-T-P for children of elementary school age: II. The "phallic tree" as an indicator of psycho-sexual conflict. *Journal of Clinical Psychology,* 1952, *8,* 245–255. (b)

Jolles, I. Child case study: The projection of a child's personality in drawings. In E.F. Hammer (Ed.), *The clinical application of projective drawings.* Springfield, IL.: Charles C. Thomas, 1958.

Jolles, I. The use of the H-T-P in a school setting. In J.N. Buck & E.F. Hammer (Eds.), *Advances in the House-Tree-Person technique: Variations and applications.* Los Angeles: Western Psychological Services, 1969.

Jolles, I. *A catalog for the qualitative interpretation of the House-Tree-Person (H-T-P)* (Rev. ed.). Los Angeles: Western Psychological Services, 1971.

Jolles, I., & Beck, H.S. A study of the validity of some hypotheses for the qualitative interpretation of the H-T-P for children of elementary school age: III. Horizontal placement. *Journal of Clinical Psychology,* 1953, *9,* 161–164. (a)

Jolles, I., & Beck, H.S. A study of the validity of some hypotheses for the qualitative intrpretation of the H-T-P for children of elementary school age: IV. Vertical placement. *Journal of Clinical Psychology,* 1953, *9,* 167. (b)

Jordan, S. Projective drawings in a cerebellar disorder due to chicken pox encephalitis. *Journal of Projective Techniques and Personality Assessment,* 1970, *34,* 256–258.

Jortner, S. An investigation of certain cognitive aspects of schizophrenia. *Journal of Projective Techniques and Personality Assessment,* 1966, *30,* 559–568.

Jortner, S. Overinclusion responses to WAIS Similarities as suggestive of schizophrenia. *Journal of Clinical Psychology,* 1970, *26,* 346–348.

Kaden, S.E., & Lipton, H. Rorschach developmental scores and post hospital adjustment of married male schizophrenics. *Journal of Projective Techniques,* 1960, *24,* 144–147.

Kadis, A. Finger painting as a projective technique. In L.E. Abt & L. Bellak (Eds.), *Projective psychology.* New York: Knopf, 1950.

Kagan, J. The long term stability of selected Rorschach responses. *Journal of Consulting Psychology,* 1960, *24,* 67–73.

Kahn, P. Time span and Rorschach human movement responses. *Journal of Consulting Psychology,* 1967, *31,* 92–93.

Kahn, T.C., & Giffen, M.B. *Psychological techniques in diagnosis and evaluation.* New York: Pergamon Press, Inc., 1960.

Kaldegg, A. Psychological observations in a group of alcoholic patients with analysis of Rorschach, Wechsler-Bellevue and Bender-Gestalt results. *Quarterly Journal of Studies in Alcoholism,* 1956, *17,* 608–628.

Kalinowsky, L.B., & Hoch, P.H. *Somatic treatments in psychiatry.* New York: Grune & Stratton, 1961.

Karlin, I.W., Eisenson, J., Hirschenfang, S., & Miller, M. A multi-evaluational study of aphasic and non-aphasic right hemiplegic patients. *Journal of Speech and Hearing Disorders,* 1959, *24,* 369–379.

Kaspar, J.C., & Schulman, J.L. Organic mental disorders: Brain damages. In B.B. Wolman (Ed.), *Manual of child psychopathology.* New York: McGraw-Hill, 1972.

Kaswan, J., Wasman, M., & Freedman, L.Z. Aggression and the picture frustration study. *Journal of Consulting Psychology,* 1960, *24,* 446–452.

Kataguchi, Y. Rorschach schizophrenic score (RSS). *Journal of Projective Techniques,* 1959, *23,* 214–222.

Kates, S.L. Objective Rorschach response patterns differentiating anxiety reactions from obsessive-compulsive reactions. *Journal of Consulting Psychology,* 1950, *14,* 226–229.

Kates, S.L., & Schwartz, F. Stress, anxiety and response complexity on the Rorschach test. *Journal of Projective Techniques,* 1958, *22,* 64–69.

Kaufman, A.S. *Intelligent testing with the WISC-R.* New York: John Wiley & Sons, Inc., 1979.

Keiser, T.W. Schizotype and the Wechsler Digit Span Test. *Journal of Clinical Psychology,* 1975, *31,* 303–306.

Keller, J.E. The use of a Bender Gestalt maturation level scoring system with mentally handicapped children. *American Journal of Orthopsychiatry,* 1955, *25,* 563–573.

Kelley, D., & Klopfer, B. Application of the Rorschach method to research in schizophrenia. *Rorschach Research Exchange,* 1939, *3,* 55–66.

Kendra, J.M. Predicting suicide using the Rorschach inkblot test. *Journal of Personality Assessment,* 1979, *43,* 452–456.

King, G.F. A theoretical and experimental consideration of the Rorschach human movement response. *Psychological Monographs,* 1958, *72* (No. 5).

King, G.F. An interpersonal conception of Rorschach human movement and delusional content. *Journal of Projective Techniques*, 1960, *24*, 161–163.

Kisker, G.W. The Rorschach analysis of psychotics subjected to neurosurgical interruption of the thalamocortical projections. *Psychiatric Quarterly*, 1944, *18*, 43–52.

Kleinman, R.A., & Higgins, J. Sex of respondent and Rorschach M production. *Journal of Projective Techniques and Personality Assessment*, 1966, *30*, 439–440.

Klopfer, B., Ainsworth, M., Klopfer, W., & Holt, R. *Developments in the Rorschach technique, Vol. I: Technique and theory*. New York: Harcourt Brace Jovanovich, 1954.

Klopfer, B., & Davidson, H. *The Rorschach technique: An introductory manual*. New York: Harcourt Brace Jovanovich, 1962.

Klopfer, B., et al. *Developments in the Rorschach technique, Vol. II: Fields of application*. New York: Harcourt Brace Jovanovich, 1956.

Klopfer, B., & Kelley, D. *The Rorschach technique*. New York: World Book, 1942.

Klopfer, W.G., & Taulbee, E.S. Projective tests. *Annual Review of Psychology*, 1976, *27*, 543–567.

Klove, H. Relationship of differential electroencephalographic patterns to distribution of Wechsler-Bellevue scores. *Neurology*, 1959, *9*, 871–876.

Klove, H. Validation studies in adult clinical neuropsychology. In R.M. Reitan & L.A. Davison (Eds.), *Clinical neuropsychology: Current status and applications*. New York: Halstead Press, 1974.

Klove, H., & Fitzhugh, K.B. The relationship of differential EEG patterns to the distribution of Wechsler-Bellevue scores in a chronic epileptic population. *Journal of Clinical Psychology*, 1962, *18*, 334–337.

Klove, H., & Reitan, R.M. Effect of dysphasia and spatial distortion on Wechsler-Bellevue results. *Archives of Neurology and Psychiatry*, 1958, *80*, 708–713.

Knopf, I.J. Rorschach summary scores in differential diagnosis. *Journal of Consulting Psychology*, 1956, *20*, 99–104.

Knopf, I.J. Rorschach summary scores in differential diagnosis. In B.I. Murstein (Ed.), *Handbook of projective techniques*. New York: Basic Books, 1965.

Koch, C. *The Tree Test*. New York: Grune & Stratton, 1952.

Kodman, F., Jr., & Waters, J. Rorschach responses of children exhibiting psychogenic auditory symptoms. *Journal of Clinical Psychology*, 1961, *17*, 305–306.

Kohn, B., & Dennis, M. Patterns of hemispheric specialization after hemidecortication for infantile hemiplegia. In M. Kinsbourne & W.L. Smith (Eds.), *Hemispheric disconnection and cerebral function*. Springfield, IL.: Charles C. Thomas, 1974.

Kokonis, N.D. Body image disturbance in schizophrenia: A study of arms and feet. *Journal of Personality Assessment*, 1972, *36*, 573–575.

Koppitz, E.M. The Bender-Gestalt Test and learning disturbances in young children. *Journal of Clinical Psychology*, 1958, *14*, 292–295.

Koppitz, E.M. The Bender Gestalt Test for children: A normative study. *Journal of Clinical Psychology*, 1960, *16*, 432–435.

Koppitz, E.M. Diagnosing brain damage in young children with the Bender-Gestalt test. *Journal of Consulting Psychology*, 1962, *26*, 541–545.

Koppitz, E.M. *The Bender Gestalt Test for young children*. New York: Grune & Stratton, 1964.

Koppitz, E.M. Emotional indicators on human figure drawings and school achievement of first and second graders. *Journal of Clinical Psychology*, 1966, *22*, 481–483. (a)

Koppitz, E.M. Emotional indicators on human figure drawings of children: A validation study. *Journal of Clinical Psychology*, 1966, *22*, 313–315. (b)

Koppitz, E.M. Emotional indicators on human figure drawings of shy and aggressive children. *Journal of Clinical Psychology*, 1966, *22*, 466–469. (c)

Koppitz, E.M. *Psychological evaluation of children's human figure drawings*. New York: Grune & Stratton, 1968.

Korchin, S.J. Form perception and ego functioning. In M. Rickers-Ovsiankina (Ed.), *Rorschach psychology*. New York: John Wiley & Sons, Inc., 1960.

Korchin, S.J., & Larson, D.G. Form perception and ego functioning. In M. Rickers-Ovsiankina (Ed.), *Rorschach psychology* (2nd ed.). New York: Krieger, 1977.

Kral, V.A., & Dorken, H. Deterioration in dementia paralytica. *American Journal of Psychiatry*, 1953, *109*, 684–692.

Krippner, S. WISC comprehension and picture arrangement subtests as measures of social competence. *Journal of Clinical Psychology*, 1964, *20*, 366–367.

Krout, J. Symbol elaboration test. *Psychological Monographs*, 1950, *64* (No. 310).

Kuhn, R. Some problems concerning the psychological implications of Rorschach's form interpretation test (J. Huttner, trans.). In M. Rickers-Ovsiankina (Ed.), *Rorschach psychology*. New York: John Wiley & Sons, Inc., 1960.

Kunce, J.T., Ryan, J.J., & Eckelman, C.C. Violent behavior and differential WAIS characteristics. *Journal of Consulting and Clinical Psychology*, 1976, *44*, 42–45.

Kurtzberg, R., Cavior, N., & Lipton, D. Sex drawn first and sex drawn larger by opiate addict and non-addict inmates on the Draw-A-Person test. *Journal of Projective Techniques and Personality Assessment*, 1966, *30*, 55–58.

Kurz, R.B. Relationship between time imagery and Rorschach human movement responses. *Journal of Consulting Psychology*, 1963, *27*, 273–276.

Kwawer, J.S. Male homosexual psychodynamics and the Rorschach test. *Journal of Personality Assessment*, 1977, *41*, 10–18.

Lacks, P.B., Harrow, M., Colbert, J., & Levine, J. Further evidence concerning the diagnostic accuracy of the Halstead organic test battery. *Journal of Clinical Psychology*, 1970, *26*, 480–481.

Ladd, C.E. WAIS performances of brain damaged and neurotic patients. *Journal of Clinical Psychology*, 1964, *20*, 114–117.

Laird, J. A comparison of male normals, psychiatric patients and alcoholics for sex drawn first. *Journal of Clinical Psychology*, 1962, *18*, 302.

Lakin, M. Certain formal characteristics of human figure drawings by institutionalized aged and by normal children. *Journal of Consulting Psychology*, 1956, *20*, 471–474.

Lambley, P. Rorschach scores and schizophrenia: An evaluation of Weiner's signs in clinical practice. *Journal of Personality Assessment*, 1973, *37*, 420–423.

Landisberg, S. Relationship of the Rorschach to projective drawings. In E.F. Hammer (Ed.), *The clinical application of projective drawings*. Springfield, IL.: Charles C. Thomas, 1958.

Landisberg, S. The use of the H-T-P in a mental hygiene clinic for children. In J.N. Buck & E.F. Hammer (Eds.), *Advances in the House-Tree-Person technique: Variations and applications*. Los Angeles: Western Psychological Services, 1969.

Lanfeld, E.S., & Saunders, D.R. Anxiety as "effect of uncertainty": An experiment illuminating the OA subtest of the WAIS. *Journal of Clinical Psychology*, 1961, *17*, 238–241.

Laughlin, H.P. *The ego and its defenses* (2nd ed.). New York: Appleton-Century-Crofts, 1979.

Lebo, D., Toal, R., & Brick, H. Rorschach performance in the amelioration and continuation of observable anxiety. *Journal of General Psychology*, 1960, *63*, 75–80.

Lehner, G.F., & Gunderson, E.K. Height relationships in DAP test. *Journal of Personality*, 1948, *17*, 199–209.

Lehner, G.F.J., & Kube, E. *The dynamics of personal adjustment*. Englewood Cliffs, N.J.: Prentice Hall, 1955.

Lerner, B. Rorschach movement and dreams: A validation study using drug-induced dream deprivation. *Journal of Abnormal Psychology*, 1966, *71*, 75–86.

Lerner, E.A. *The projective use of the Bender Gestalt*. Springfield, IL.: Charles C. Thomas, 1972.

Lerner, J., & Shanan, J. Coping style of psychiatric patients with somatic complaints. *Journal of Personality Assessment*, 1972, *36*, 28–32.

Lester, D., Kendra, J.M., Thisted, R.A., & Perdue, W.C. Prediction of homicide with the Rorschach. *Journal of Clinical Psychology*, 1975, *31*, 752.

Lester, D., & Perdue, W.C. Suicide, homicide, and color-shading response on the Rorschach. *Perceptual and Motor Skills*, 1972, *35*, 562.

Levenson, M. Cognitive correlates of suicidal risk. In C. Neuringer (Ed.), *Psychological assessment of suicide risk*. Springfield, IL.: Charles C. Thomas, 1974.

Levenson, M., & Neuringer, C. Problem-solving behavior in suicidal adolescents. *Journal of Consulting and Clinical Psychology*, 1971, *37*, 433–436.

Levi, J. Rorschach patterns predicting success or failure in rehabilitation of the physically handicapped. *Journal of Abnormal and Social Psychology*, 1951, *46*, 240–244.

Levi, J. Acting out indicators on the Rorschach. In L. Abt & S. Weissman (Eds.), *Acting out*. New York: Grune & Stratton, 1965.

Levi, J., Oppenheim, S., & Wechsler, D. Clinical use of the Mental Deterioration Index of the Bellevue-Wechsler Scale. *Journal of Abnormal and Social Psychology*, 1945, *40*, 405–407.

Levine, A., & Sapolsky, A. The use of the H-T-P as an aid in the screening of hospitalized patients. In J.N. Buck and E.F. Hammer (Eds.), *Advances in the House-Tree-Person technique: Variations and applications*. Los Angeles: Western Psychological Services, 1969.

Levine, J., & Feirstein, A. Differences in test performance between brain-damaged, schizophrenic, and medical patients. *Journal of Consulting and Clinical Psychology*, 1972, *39*, 508–511.

Levine, M., Glass, H., & Meltzoff, J. The inhibition process, Rorschach movement responses, and intelligence. *Journal of Consulting Psychology*, 1957, *21*, 41–45.

Levine, M., & Meltzoff, J. Cognitive inhibition and Rorschach human movement responses. *Journal of Consulting Psychology*, 1956, *20*, 119–122.

Levine, M., & Spivack, G. Human movement responses and verbal expression in the Rorschach test. *Journal of Projective Techniques*, 1962, *26*, 299–304.

Levine, M., & Spivack, G. *The Rorschach index of repressive style*. Springfield, IL.: Charles C. Thomas, 1964.

Levitt, E.E. Alleged Rorschach anxiety indices in children. *Journal of Projective Techniques*, 1957, *21*, 261–264.

Levitt, E., & Grosz, H. A comparison of quantifiable Rorschach anxiety indicators in hypnotically induced anxiety states. *Journal of Consulting Psychology*, 1960, *24*, 31–34.

Levitt, E., Lubin, B., & Zuckerman, M. A simplified method of scoring Rorschach content for dependency. *Journal of Projective Techniques*, 1962, *26*, 234–236.

Levitt, E., & Truumaa, A. *The Rorschach technique with children and adolescents: Application and norms*. New York: Grune & Stratton, 1972.

Levy, S. Figure drawing as a projective test. In L.E. Abt & L. Bellak (Eds.), *Projective psychology*. New York: Knopf, 1950.

Levy, S. Projective figure drawing. In E.F. Hammer (Ed.), *The clinical application of projective drawings*. Springfield, IL.: Charles C. Thomas, 1958.

Lewandowski, N.G., Saccuzzo, D.P., & Lewandowski, D.G. The WISC as a measure of personality types. *Journal of Clinical Psychology*, 1977, *33*, 285–291.

Lewinski, R.J. The psychometric pattern: I. Anxiety neurosis. *Journal of Clinical Psychology*, 1945, *1*, 214–221.

Lewinski, R.J. The psychometric pattern: III. Epilepsy. *American Journal of Orthopsychiatry*, 1947, *17*, 714–722.

Lewinsohn, P.M. Relationship between height of figure drawings and depression in psychiatric patients. *Journal of Consulting Psychology*, 1964, *28*, 380–381.

Lezak, M. *Neuropsychological assessment*. New York: Oxford University Press, 1976.

Lindner, R.M. Content analysis in Rorschach work. *Rorschach Research Exchange*, 1946, *10*, 121–129.

Lindner, R.M. Analysis of the Rorschach test by content. *Journal of Clinical Psychopathology*, 1947, *8*, 707–719.

Lindner, R.M. The content analysis of the Rorschach protocol. In L.E. Abt & L. Bellak (Eds.), *Projective psychology*. New York: Knopf, 1950.

Lord, E. Experimentally induced variations in Rorschach performance. *Psychological Monographs*, 1950, *64* (No. 316).

Lubin, B., Wallis, R.R., & Paine, C. Patterns of psychological test usage in the United States: 1935–1969. *Professional Psychology*, 1971, *2*, 70–74.

Lucas, W. The effects of frustration on the Rorschach responses of nine year old children. *Journal of Projective Techniques*, 1961, *25*, 199–204.

Ludwig, D.J. Self-perception and the Draw-a-Person Test. *Journal of Projective Techniques and Personality Assessment*, 1969, *33*, 257–261.

Luria, A.R. Psychological studies of mental deficiency in the Soviet Union. In N.R. Ellis (Ed.), *Handbook of mental deficiency*. New York: McGraw-Hill, 1963.

Luria, A.R. Neuropsychology in the local diagnosis of brain damage. *Cortex*, 1964, *1*, 3–18.

Mabry, M. Serial projective drawings in a patient with a malignant brain tumor. *Journal of Projective Techniques*, 1964, *28*, 206–209.

Machover, K. *Personality projection in the drawing of the human figure*. Springfield, IL.: Charles C. Thomas, 1949.

Machover, K. Drawings of the human figure: A method of personality investigation. In H.H. Anderson & G. Anderson (Eds.), *An introduction to projective techniques*. Englewood Cliffs, N.J.: Prentice-Hall, 1951.

Machover, K. The body image in art communication as seen in William Steig's drawings. *Journal of Projective Techniques*, 1955, *19*, 453–460.

Machover, K. Adolescent case study: A disturbed adolescent girl. In E.F. Hammer (Ed.), *The clinical application of projective drawings*. Springfield, IL.: Charles C. Thomas, 1958.

Machover, K. Sex differences in the developmental pattern of children seen in Human Figure Drawings. In A.I. Rabin & M. Haworth (Eds.), *Projective techniques with children*. New York: Grune & Stratton, 1960.

Magaret, A. Parallels in the behavior of schizophrenics, paretics, and pre-senile non-psychotics. *Journal of Abnormal and Social Psychology*, 1942, *37*, 511–528.

Maley, R.F. The relationship of premorbid social activity level of psychiatric patients to test performance on the WAIS and the MMPI. *Journal of Clinical Psychology*, 1970, *26*, 75–76.

Maloney, M.P., & Ward, M.P. *Psychological assessment*. New York: Oxford University Press, 1976.

Mandler, G., & Sarason, S.B. Anxiety as a factor in test performance. *American Psychologist*, 1951, *6*, 341.

Mann, L. The relation of Rorschach indices of extratension and introversion to a measure of responsiveness to the immediate environment. *Journal of Consulting Psychology*, 1956, *20*, 114–118.

Manne, S.H., Kandel, A., & Rosenthal, D. Differences between Performance IQ and Verbal IQ in a severely sociopathic population. *Journal of Clinical Psychology*, 1962, *18*, 73–77.

Mark, J., & Morrow, R. The use of the Bender-Gestalt Test in the study of brain damage. *American Psychologist*, 1955, *10*, 323. (Abstract)

Martin, B. *Abnormal psychology*. New York: Holt, Rinehart & Winston, 1977.

Marzolf, S.S., & Kirchner, J.H. House-Tree-Person drawings and personality traits. *Journal of Personality Assessment*, 1972, *36*, 148–165.

Masling, J., Rabie, L., & Blondheim, S. Obesity, level of aspiration, and Rorschach and TAT measures of oral dependence. *Journal of Consulting Psychology*, 1967, *31*, 233–239.

Matthews, C.G., Shaw, D.J., & Klove, H. Psychological test performances in neurologic and "pseudo-neurologic" subjects. *Cortex*, 1966, *2*, 244–253.

Mayman, M. Reality contact, defense effectiveness, and psychopathology in Rorschach form-level scores. In B. Klopfer et al. (Eds.), *Developments in the Rorschach technique, Vol. III: Aspects of Personality Structure*. New York: Harcourt Brace Jovanovich, 1970.

Mayman, M. A multi-dimensional view of the Rorschach movement response. In M. Rickers-Ovsiankina (Ed.), *Rorschach psychology* (2nd ed.). New York: Kreiger, 1977.

Mayman, M., & Cole, J. Diagnosing neurotic disorders. In B.B. Wolman (Ed.), *Clinical diagnosis of mental disorders: A handbook*. New York: Plenum Publishing Corp., 1978.

Mayman, M., Schafer, R., & Rapaport, D. Interpretation of the Wechsler-Bellevue Intelligence Scale in personality appraisal. In H.H. Anderson & G. Anderson (Eds.), *An introduction to projective techniques*. New York: Prentice-Hall, 1951.

McCue, K., Rothenberg, D., Allen, R., & Jennings, T. Rorschach variables in two "Study of Values" types. *Journal of General Psychology*, 1963, *68*, 169–172.

McCully, R.S. Human movement in the Rorschach materials of a group of pre-adolescent boys suffering from progressive muscular loss. *Journal of Projective Techniques*, 1961, *25*, 205–211.

McCully, R.S. *Rorschach theory and symbolism.* Baltimore: Williams & Wilkins, 1971.

McCully, R.S., Glucksman, M.L., & Hirsch, J. Nutrition imagery in the Rorschach materials of food-deprived, obese patients. *Journal of Projective Techniques and Personality Assessment,* 1968, *32,* 375–382.

McElhaney, M. *Clinical psychological assessment of the human figure drawing.* Springfield, IL.: Charles C. Thomas, 1969.

McFie, J. Psychological testing in clinical neurology. *Journal of Nervous and Mental Disease,* 1960, *131,* 383–393.

McFie, J. *Assessment of organic impairment.* New York: Academic Press, 1975.

McFie, J., & Thompson, J.A. Picture Arrangement: A measure of frontal lobe function? *British Journal of Psychiatry,* 1972, *121,* 547–552.

McFie, J., & Zangwill, O.L. Visual-constructive disabilities associated with lesions of the left cerebral hemisphere. *Brain,* 1960, *83,* 243–260.

McHugh, A. Children's figure drawings in neurotic and conduct disturbances. *Journal of Clinical Psychology,* 1966, *22,* 219–221.

Meier, M.J. Some challenges for clinical neuropsychology. In R.M. Reitan & L.A. Davison (Eds.), *Clinical neuropsychology: Current status and applications.* New York: Halstead Press, 1974.

Meier, M.J., & French, L.A. Lateralized deficits in complex visual discrimination and bilateral transfer of reminiscence following unilateral temporal lobectomy. *Neuropsychologia,* 1965, *3,* 261–273.

Meltzoff, J., & Levine, M. The relationship between motor and cognitive inhibition. *Journal of Consulting Psychology,* 1954, *18,* 355–358.

Meltzoff, J., & Litwin, D. Affective control and Rorschach human movement responses. *Journal of Consulting Psychology,* 1956, *20,* 463–465.

Meltzoff, J., Singer, J., & Korchin, S. Motor inhibition and Rorschach human movement responses: A test of the sensory tonic theory. *Journal of Personality,* 1953, *21,* 400–410.

Meyer, B.C., Brown, F., & Levine, A. Observations on the House-Tree-Person drawing test before and after surgery. *Psychosomatic Medicine,* 1955, *17,* 428–454.

Meyer, M.M. The case of El: Blind analysis of the tests of an unknown patient. *Journal of Projective Techniques,* 1961, *25,* 375–382.

Meyer, M.M., & Caruth, E. Rorschach indices of ego processes. In B. Klopfer et al. (Eds.), *Developments in the Rorschach technique, Vol. III: Aspects of Personality Structure.* New York: Harcourt Brace Jovanovich, 1970.

Meyer, V., & Jones, H.G. Patterns of cognitive test performance as functions of the lateral localization of cerebral abnormalities in the temporal lobe. *Journal of Mental Science,* 1957, *103,* 758–772.

Miale, F. Rorschach sequence analysis in a case of paranoid schizophrenia. *Journal of Projective Techniques,* 1947, *11,* 3–22.

Miale, F. Symbolic imagery in Rorschach material. In M. Rickers-Ovsiankina (Ed.), *Rorschach psychology* (2nd ed.). New York: Krieger, 1977.

Miale, F., & Harrower-Erickson, M. Personality structure in the psychoneuroses. *Rorschach Research Exchange,* 1940, *4,* 71–74.

Michal-Smith, H. The identification of pathological cerebral function through the H-T-P technique. *Journal of Clinical Psychology,* 1953, *9,* 293–295.

Michal-Smith, H., & Morgenstern, M. The use of the H-T-P with the mentally retarded child in a hospital clinic. In J.N. Buck & E.F. Hammer (Eds.), *Advances in the House-Tree-Person technique: Variations and applications.* Los Angeles: Western Psychological Services, 1969.

Milberg, W., Greiffenstein, M., Lewis, R., & Rourke, D. Differentiation of temporal lobe and generalized seizure patients with the WAIS. *Journal of Consulting and Clinical Psychology,* 1980, *48,* 39–42.

Modell, A.H. Changes in human figure drawings by patients who recover from regressed states. *American Journal of Orthopsychiatry,* 1951, *21,* 584–596.

Modell, A.H., & Potter, H.W. Human figure drawing of patients with arterial hypertension, peptic ulcer, and bronchial asthma. *Psychosomatic Medicine,* 1949, *11,* 282–292.

Mogar, R.E. Anxiety indices in human figure drawings. *Journal of Consulting Psychology,* 1962, *26,* 108.

Moldawsky, S., & Moldawsky, P.C. Digit span as an anxiety indicator. *Journal of Consulting Psychology,* 1952, *16,* 115–118.

Molish, H.B. The popular response in Rorschach records of normals, neurotics, and schizophrenics. *American Journal of Orthopsychiatry,* 1951, *21,* 523–531.

Molish, H.B. Critique and problems of research. A survey. In S.J. Beck & H.B. Molish, *Rorschach's test II. A variety of personality pictures.* New York: Grune & Stratton, 1967.

Mons, W.E.R. *Principles and practice of the Rorschach personality test.* London: Faber & Faber, 1950.

Montague, D.J., & Prytula, R.E. Human figure drawing characteristics related to juvenile delinquents. *Perceptual and Motor Skills,* 1975, *40,* 623–630.

Morrow, R.S., & Mark, J.C. The correlation of intelligence and neurological findings on twenty-two patients autopsied for brain damage. *Journal of Consulting Psychology,* 1955, *19,* 283–289.

Mosher, D.L., & Smith J.P. The usefulness of two scoring systems for the Bender Gestalt Test for identifying brain damage. *Journal of Consulting Psychology,* 1965, *29,* 530–536.

Moylan, J.J., Shaw, J., & Appleman, W. Passive and aggressive responses to the Rorschach by passive-aggressive personalities and paranoid schizophrenics. *Journal of Projective Techniques,* 1960, *24,* 17–20.

Mukerji, M. Rorschach indices of love, aggression and happiness. *Journal of Projective Techniques and Personality Assessment*, 1969, *33*, 526–529.

Mundy, J. The use of projective techniques with children. In B.B. Wolman (Ed.), *Manual of child psychopathology*. New York: McGraw-Hill, 1972.

Munroe, R. Prediction of the adjustment and academic performance of college students by a modification of the Rorschach method. *Applied Psychological Monographs*, 1945 (No 7).

Munroe, R. The inspection technique for the Rorschach protocol. In L.E. Abt & L. Bellak (Eds.), *Projective psychology*. New York: Knopf, 1950.

Murray, E., & Roberts, F. The Bender-Gestalt Test in a patient passing through a brief manic-depressive cycle. *U.S. Armed Forces Medical Journal*, 1956, *7*, 1206–1208.

Mursell, G.R. The use of the H-T-P with the mentally deficient. In J.N. Buck & E.F. Hammer (Eds.), *Advances in the House-Tree-Person technique: Variations and applications*. Los Angeles: Western Psychological Services, 1969.

Murstein, B.I. Personality and intellectual changes in leukemia: A case study. *Journal of Projective Techniques*, 1958, *22*, 421–426.

Murstein, B.I. Factor analysis of the Rorschach. *Journal of Consulting Psychology*, 1960, *24*, 262–275.

Neel, A. Inhibition and perception of movement on the Rorschach. *Journal of Consulting Psychology*, 1960, *24*, 224–230.

Neiger, S., Slemon, A., & Quirk, D. The performance of chronic schizophrenic patients on Piotrowski's Rorschach sign list for CNS pathology. *Journal of Projective Techniques*, 1962, *26*, 419–428.

Neuringer, C. Manifestations of anxiety on the Rorschach Test. *Journal of Projective Techniques*, 1962, *26*, 318–326.

Neuringer, C. Rorschach inkblot test assessment of suicidal risk. In C. Neuringer (Ed.), *Psychological assessment of suicidal risk*. Springfield, IL.: Charles C. Thomas, 1974.

Newmark, C.S., Finkelstein, M., & Frerking, R.A. Comparison of the predictive validity of two measures of psychotherapy prognosis. *Journal of Personality Assessment*, 1974, *38*, 144–148.

Newmark, C.S., Hetzel, W., Walker, L., Holstein, S., & Finkelstein, M. Predictive validity of the Rorschach Prognostic Rating Scale with behavior modification techniques. *Journal of Clinical Psychology*, 1973, *29*, 246–248.

Nickerson, E.T. Some correlates of M. *Journal of Projective Techniques and Personality Assessment*, 1969, *33*, 203–212.

Norman, R.P., & Wilensky, H. Item difficulty of the WAIS Information subtest for a chronic schizophrenic sample. *Journal of Clinical Psychology*, 1961, *17*, 56–57.

Ogdon, D.P. *Psychodiagnostics and personality assessment: A handbook* (2nd ed.). Los Angeles: Western Psychological Services, 1975.

Olch, D.R. Psychometric patterns of schizophrenics on the Wechsler-Bellevue Intelligence Test. *Journal of Consulting Psychology*, 1948, *12*, 127–136.

Olch, D. Personality characteristics of hemophiliacs. *Journal of Personality Assessment*, 1971, *35*, 72–79.

O'Leary, M.R., Donovan, D.M., Chaney, E.F., Walker, R.D., & Shau, E.J. Application of discriminant analysis to level of performance of alcoholics and nonalcoholics on Wechsler-Bellevue and Halstead-Reitan subtests. *Journal of Clinical Psychology*, 1979, *35*, 204–208.

Orme, J.E. The Rorschach sex response in a psychiatric population. *Journal of Clinical Psychology*, 1962, *18*, 303.

Orme, J.E. Rorschach alphabetical and geometrical responses. *Journal of Clinical Psychology*, 1963, *19*, 459–460.

Orme, J.E. A study of Weiner's Rorschach indicators. *Journal of Clinical Psychology*, 1964, *20*, 531–532.

Orme, J.E. A further comment on Weiner's Rorschach color indicators. *Journal of Clinical Psychology*, 1966, *22*, 223.

Overall, J.E., & Gorham, D.R. Organicity versus old age in objective and projective test performance. *Journal of Consulting and Clinical Psychology*, 1972, *39*, 98–105.

Overall, J.E., Hoffmann, N.G., & Levin, H. Effects of aging, organicity, alcoholism, and functional psychopathology on WAIS subtest profiles. *Journal of Consulting and Clinical Psychology*, 1978, *46*, 1315–1322.

Page, H.A. Studies in fantasy-daydreaming frequency and Rorschach scoring categories. *Journal of Consulting Psychology*, 1957, *21*, 111–114.

Palmer, J.O. *The psychological assessment of children*. New York: John Wiley & Sons, Inc., 1970.

Palmer, J.O., & Lustgarten, B.J. The prediction of TAT structure as a test of Rorschach's experience-balance. *Journal of Projective Techniques*, 1962, *26*, 212–220.

Panton, J.H. Beta-WAIS comparison and WAIS subtest configurations within a state prison population. *Journal of Clinical Psychology*, 1960, *16*, 312–317.

Papanek, E. Management of acting out adolescents. In L.E. Abt & S.L. Weissman (Eds.), *Acting out*. New York: Grune & Stratton, 1965.

Parker, J.W. The validity of some current tests for organicity. *Journal of Consulting Psychology*, 1957, *21*, 425–428.

Parsons, O.A., Morris, F., & Denny, J.P. Agitation, anxiety, brain damage and perceptual-motor deficit. *Journal of Clinical Psychology*, 1963, *19*, 267–271.

Parsons, O.A., Vega, A., & Burn, J. Different psychological effects of lateralized brain-damage. *Journal of Consulting and Clinical Psychology*, 1969, *33*, 551–557.

Pascal, G.R., Ruesch, H.A., Devine, C.A., & Suttell, B. A study of genital symbols on the Rorschach test. *Journal of Abnormal and Social Psychology*, 1950, *45*, 286–295.

Pascal, G.R., & Suttell, B. *The Bender-Gestalt Test*. New York: Grune & Stratton, 1951.

Patterson, C.H. *The Wechsler-Bellevue Scales: A guide for counselors*. Springfield, IL.: Charles C. Thomas, 1953.

Payne, J.J. Comments on the analysis of chromatic drawings. *Journal of Clinical Psychology*, 1948, *5*, 119–120. (Monograph Supplement)

Peek, R.M. Directionality of lines in the Bender-Gestalt Test. *Journal of Consulting Psychology*, 1953, *17*, 213–216.

Perdue, W.C. Rorschach responses of 100 murderers. *Corrective Psychiatry and Journal of Social Therapy*, 1964, *10* (No. 6).

Philippus, M.J. Atypical diagnostic conditions. In W.L. Smith & M.J. Philippus (Eds.), *Neuropsychological testing in organic brain dysfunction*. Springfield, IL.: Charles C. Thomas, 1969.

Phillips, L., & Smith, J. *Rorschach interpretation: Advanced technique*. New York: Grune & Stratton, 1953.

Pierce, D., Cooke, G., & Frahm, P. Sort-score correlates of schizophrenia. *Journal of Personality Assessment*, 1973, *37*, 508–511.

Piotrowski, Z. The M, FM, and m responses as indicators of changes in personality. *Rorschach Research Exchange*, 1937, *1*, 148–156. (a)

Piotrowski, Z. The Rorschach inkblot method in organic disturbances of the central nervous system. *Journal of Nervous and Mental Disease*, 1937, *86*, 525–537. (b)

Piotrowski, Z. *Perceptanalysis*. New York: Macmillan, 1957.

Piotrowski, Z. The movement score. In M. Rickers-Ovsiankina (Ed.), *Rorschach psychology*. New York: John Wiley & Sons, Inc., 1960.

Piotrowski, Z. Long-term prognosis in schizophrenia based on Rorschach findings: The LTPTI. In D.V. Siva Sankar (Ed.), *Schizophrenia: Current concepts and research*. Hicksville, N.Y.: PJD Publications, 1969.

Piotrowski, Z. The movement responses. In M. Rickers-Ovsiankina (Ed.), *Rorschach psychology* (2nd ed.). New York: Kreiger, 1977.

Piotrowski, Z., & Berg, D.A. Verification of the Rorschach Alpha diagnostic formula for underactive schizophrenics. *American Journal of Psychiatry*, 1955, *112*, 443–450.

Piotrowski, Z., & Bricklin, B. A second validation of a long-term Rorschach prognostic index for schizophrenic patients. *Journal of Consulting Psychology*, 1961, *25*, 123–128.

Piotrowski, Z., & Dudek, S. Research on human movement response in the Rorschach examinations of marital partners. In V.W. Eisenstein (Ed.), *Neurotic interaction in marriage*. New York: Basic Books, 1956.

Piotrowski, Z., & Levine, D. A case illustrating the concept of the alpha schizophrenic. *Journal of Projective Techniques*, 1959, *23*, 223–236.

Piotrowski, Z., & Lewis, N.D.C. An experimental Rorschach diagnostic aid for some forms of schizophrenia. *American Journal of Psychiatry*, 1950, *107*, 360–366.

Pollitt, E., Hirsch, S., & Money, J. Priapism, impotence and human figure drawing. *Journal of Nervous and Mental Disease*, 1964, *139*, 161–168.

Pope, B., & Scott, W.H. *Psychological diagnosis in clinical practice*. New York: Oxford University Press, 1967.

Potkay, C.R. *The Rorschach clinician*. New York: Grune & Stratton, 1971.

Powers, W.T., & Hamlin, R.M. Relationship between diagnostic category and defiant verbalizations on the Rorschach. *Journal of Consulting Psychology*, 1955, *19*, 120–124.

Prandoni, J.R., Jensen, D.E., Matranga, J.T., & Waison, M.O.S. Selected Rorschach response characteristics of sex offenders. *Journal of Personality Assessment*, 1973, *37*, 334–336.

Precker, J.A. Painting and drawing in personality assessment. *Journal of Projective Techniques*, 1950, *14*, 262-286.

Prentice, N.M., & Kelly, F.J. Intelligence and delinquency: A reconsideration. *Journal of Social Psychology*, 1963, *60*, 327–337.

Quast, W. The Bender-Gestalt: A clinical study of children's records. *Journal of Consulting Psychology*, 1961, *25*, 405–408.

Quinlan, D.M., & Harrow, M. Boundary disturbances in schizophrenia. *Journal of Abnormal Psychology*, 1974, *83*, 533–541.

Quinlan, D.M., Harrow, M., Tucker, G., & Carlson, K. Varieties of "disordered" thinking on the Rorschach: Findings in schizophrenic and nonschizophrenic patients. *Journal of Abnormal Psychology*, 1972, *79*, 47–53.

Quirk, D., Quarrington, M., Neiger, S., & Slemon, A. The performance of acute psychotic patients on the Index of Pathological Thinking and on selected signs of idiosyncrasy on the Rorschach. *Journal of Projective Techniques*, 1962, *26*, 431–441.

Rabin, A.I. Test score patterns in schizophrenia and non-psychotic states. *Journal of Psychology*, 1941, *12*, 90–100.

Rabin, A.I. Differentiating psychometric patterns in schizophrenia and manic-depressive psychosis. *Journal of Abnormal and Social Psychology*, 1942, *37*, 270–272.

Rabin, A.I. Homicide and attempted suicide: A Rorschach study. *American Journal of Orthopsychiatry*, 1946, *16*, 516–524.

Rabin, A.I., & Hayes, D.L. Concerning the rationale of diagnostic testing. In B.B. Wolman (Ed.), *Clinical diagnosis of mental disorders: A handbook*. New York: Plenum Publishing Corp., 1978.

Rabin, A.I., & McKinney, J.P. Intelligence tests and childhood psychopathology. In B.B. Wolman (Ed.), *Manual of child psychopathology*. New York: McGraw-Hill, 1972.

Rachman, S.J., & Hodgson, R.J. *Obsessions and compulsions*. New York: Prentice-Hall, 1980.

Rader, G.E. The prediction of overt aggressive verbal behavior from Rorschach content. *Journal of Projective Techniques*, 1957, *21*, 294–306.

Raifman, I. Rorschach findings in a group of peptic ulcer patients and two control groups. *Journal of Projective Techniques*, 1957, *21*, 307–312.

Rapaport, D., Gill, M., & Schafer, R. *Diagnostic psychological testing* (Vol. I). Chicago: Year Book Publishers, 1945.

Rapaport, D., Gill, M., & Schafer, R. *Diagnostic psychological testing* (Vol. II). Chicago: Year Book Publishers, 1946.

Rappaport, S.R. Intellectual deficit in organics and schizophrenics. *Journal of Consulting Psychology*, 1953, *17*, 389–395.

Rashkis, H.A., & Welsh, G.S. Detection of anxiety by use of the Wechsler scale. *Journal of Clinical Psychology*, 1946, *2*, 354–357.

Rav, J. Anatomy responses in the Rorschach test. *Journal of Projective Techniques*, 1951, *15*, 433–443.

Reed, H.B.C., Jr., & Reitan, R.M. Intelligence test performances of brain damaged subjects with lateralized motor deficits. *Journal of Consulting Psychology*, 1963, *27*, 102–106.

Reisman, J.M. An interpretation of m. *Journal of Consulting Psychology*, 1961, *25*, 367.

Reitan, R.M. Certain differential effects of left and right cerebral lesions in human adults. *Journal of Comparative and Physiological Psychology*, 1955, *48*, 474–477. (a)

Reitan, R.M. Discussion: Symposium on the temporal lobe. *Archives of Neurology and Psychiatry*, 1955, *74*, 569–570. (b)

Reitan, R.M. Validity of Rorschach test as measure of psychological effects of brain damage. *Archives of Neurology and Psychiatry*, 1955, *73*, 445–451. (c)

Reitan, R.M. Psychological deficit. *Annual Review of Psychology*, 1962, *13*, 415–444.

Reitan, R.M. Psychological deficits resulting from cerebral lesions in man. In J.M. Warren & K. Akert (Eds.), *Prefrontal grannular cortex and behavior*. New York: McGraw-Hill, 1964.

Reitan, R.M. Psychological assessment of deficits associated with brain lesions in subjects with normal and subnormal intelligence. In J.L. Khanna (Ed.), *Brain damage and mental retardation*. Springfield, IL.: Charles C. Thomas, 1967.

Reitan, R.M. Methodological problems in clinical neuropsychology. In R.M. Reitan & L.A. Davison (Eds.), *Clinical neuropsychology: Current status and applications*. New York: Halstead Press, 1974.

Reitan, R.M., & Davison, L.A. *Clinical neuropsychology: Current status and applications*. New York: Halstead Press, 1974.

Reitan, R.M., & Reed, H.B.C., Jr. Consistencies in Wechsler-Bellevue mean values in brain damaged groups. *Perceptual and Motor Skills*, 1962, *15*, 119–121.

Reitzell, J.M. A comparative study of hysterics, homosexuals and alcoholics using content analysis of Rorschach responses. *Rorschach Research Exchange and Journal of Projective Techniques*, 1949, *13*, 127–141.

Reynolds, C.R. A quick scoring guide to the interpretation of children's kinetic family drawings. *Psychology in the Schools*, 1978, *15*, 489–492.

Reznikoff, M., & Nicholas, A. An evaluation of human-figure drawing indicators of paranoid pathology. *Journal of Consulting Psychology*, 1958, *22*, 395–397.

Reznikoff, M., & Tomblen, D. The use of human figure drawings in the diagnosis of organic pathology. *Journal of Consulting Psychology*, 1956, *20*, 467–470.

Rickers-Ovsiankina, M. Longitudinal approach to schizophrenia through the Rorschach method. *Journal of Clinical Experimental Psychopathology*, 1954, *15*, 107–118.

Rickers-Ovsiankina, M. Synopsis of psychological premises underlying the Rorschach. In M. Rickers-Ovsiankina (Ed.), *Rorschach psychology*. New York: John Wiley & Sons, Inc., 1960.

Rierdan, J., Lang, E., & Eddy, S. Suicide and transparency responses on the Rorschach: A replication. *Journal of Consulting and Clinical Psychology*, 1978, *46*, 1162–1163.

Ries, H.A., Johnson, M.H., Armstrong, H., & Holmes, D.S. The draw-a-person test and process reactive schizophrenia. *Journal of Projective Techniques and Personality Assessment*, 1966, *30*, 184–186.

Riessman, F., & Miller, S.M. Social class and projective tests. *Journal of Projective Techniques*, 1958, *22*, 432–439.

Riklan, M., Zahn, T., & Diller, L. Human figure drawings before and after chemosurgery of the basal ganglia in Parkinsonism. *Journal of Nervous and Mental Disease*, 1962, *135*, 500–506.

Ritzler, B., Zambianco, D., Harder, D., & Kaskey, M. Psychotic patterns of the concept of the object on the Rorschach test. *Journal of Abnormal Psychology*, 1980, *89*, 46–55.

Roback, H.B. Human figure drawings: Their utility in the clinical psychologist's armamentarium for personality assessment. *Psychological Bulletin*, 1968, *70*, 1–19.

Roback, H., & Webersinn, A. Size of figure drawings of depressed psychiatric patients. *Journal of Abnormal Psychology*, 1966, *71*, 416.

Rorschach, H. *Psychodiagnostik* (P. Lemkau & B. Kronenberg, trans.). Bern: Huber, 1951. (Originally published, 1921.)

Rosenzweig, S., & Kogan, K. *Psychodiagnosis*. New York: Grune & Stratton, 1949.

Ross, W.D. Anatomical perseveration in Rorschach records. *Rorschach Research Exchange*, 1940, *4*, 138–145.

Ross, W.D., & Ross, S. Some Rorschach ratings of clinical value. *Rorschach Research Exchange*, 1944, *8*, 1–9.

Rossi, A., & Neuman, G. A comparative study of Rorschach norms: Medical students. *Journal of Projective Techniques*, 1961, *25*, 334–338.

Russell, E.W. WAIS factor analysis with brain damaged subjects using criterion measures. *Journal of Consulting and Clinical Psychology*, 1972, *39*, 133–139.

Russell, E.W. Three patterns of brain damage on the WAIS. *Journal of Clinical Psychology*, 1979, *35*, 611–620.

Russell, E.W., Neuringer, C., & Goldstein, G. *Assessment of brain damage*. New York: John Wiley & Sons, Inc., 1970.

Rychlak, J.F. Forced associations, symbolism, and Rorschach constructs. *Journal of Consulting Psychology*, 1959, *23*, 455–460.

Rychlak, J.F., & Guinouard, D.E. Symbolic interpretation of Rorschach content. *Journal of Consulting Psychology*, 1961, *25*, 370–380.

Rycroft, C. *A critical dictionary of psychoanalysis*. Totowa, N.J.: Littlefield, Adams & Co., 1973.

Saarni, C., & Azara, V. Developmental analysis of human figure drawings in adolescence, young adulthood, and middle age. *Journal of Personality Assessment*, 1977, *41*, 31–38.

Saccuzzo, D.P., & Lewandowski, D.G. The WISC as a diagnostic tool. *Journal of Clinical Psychology*, 1976, *32*, 115–124.

Sakheim, G.A. Suicidal responses on the Rorschach test: A validation study. Protocols of suicidal mental hospital patients compared with those of non-suicidal patients. *Journal of Nervous and Mental Disease*, 1955, *122*, 332–344.

Sandler, J., & Ackner, B. Rorschach content analysis: An experimental investigation. *British Journal of Medical Psychology*, 1951, *24*, 180–201.

Santostefano, S., & Baker, A.H. The contribution to developmental psychology. In B.B. Wolman (Ed.), *Manual of child psychopathology*. New York: McGraw-Hill, 1972.

Sapolsky, A. An indicator of suicidal ideation on the Rorschach test. *Journal of Projective Techniques*, 1963, *27*, 332–335.

Sarason, S.B. *The clinical interaction*. New York: Harper & Row, 1954.

Sattler, J.M. *Assessment of children's intelligence*. Philadelphia: Saunders, 1974.

Satz, P. Specific and nonspecific effects of brain lesions in man. *Journal of Abnormal Psychology*, 1966, *71*, 65–70.

Satz, P., Richard, W., & Daniels, A. The alteration of intellectual performance after lateralized brain-injury in man. *Psychonomic Science*, 1967, *7*, 369–370.

Schachtel, E.G. On color and affect. *Psychiatry*, 1943, *6*, 393–409.

Schachtel, E.G. *Experiential foundations of Rorschach's test*. New York: Basic Books, 1966.

Schaeffer, D.S. Scores on neuroticism pathology, mood, and Rorschach and diagnosis of affective disorder. *Psychological Reports*, 1977, *40*, 1135–1141.

Schafer, R. *Clinical application of psychological tests*. New York: International Universities Press, 1948.

Schafer, R. *Psychoanalytic interpretation in Rorschach testing*. New York: Grune & Stratton, 1954.

Schafer, R. Bodies in schizophrenic Rorschach responses. *Journal of Projective Techniques*, 1960, *24*, 267–281.

Schildkrout, M.S., Shenker, I.R., and Sonnenblick, M. *Human figure drawings in adolescence*. New York: Brunner/Mazel, 1972.

Schlesinger, L.B. Rorschach human movement responses of acting-out and withdrawn adolescents. *Perceptual and Motor Skills*, 1978, *47*, 68–70.

Schneider, M.A., & Spivack, G. An investigative study of the Bender-Gestalt: Clinical validation of its use with a reading disabled population. *Journal of Clinical Psychology*, 1979, *35*, 346–351.

Schwartz, F., & Kates, S. Rorschach performance, anxiety level, and stress. *Journal of Projective Techniques*, 1957, *21*, 154–160.

Schwartz, S., & Giacoman, S. Convergent and discriminant validity of three measures of adjustment and three measures of social desirability. *Journal of Consulting and Clinical Psychology*, 1972, *39*, 239–242.

Shapiro, D. A perceptual understanding of color response. In M. Rickers-Ovsiankina (Ed.), *Rorschach psychology*. New York: John Wiley & Sons, Inc. 1960.

Shapiro, D. A perceptual understanding of color response. In M. Rickers-Ovsiankina (Ed.), *Rorschach psychology* (2nd ed.). New York: Krieger, 1977.

Shapiro, M.B., Field, J., & Post, F. An enquiry into the determinants of a differentiation between elderly "organic" and "non-organic" psychiatric patients on the Bender Gestalt Test. *Journal of Mental Science*, 1957, *103*, 364–374.

Shatin, L. Psychoneurosis and psychosomatic reactions: A Rorschach contrast. *Journal of Consulting Psychology*, 1952, *16*, 220–223.

Shaw, M.C., & Cruickshank, W. The Rorschach performance of epileptic children. *Journal of Consulting Psychology*, 1957, *21*, 422–424.

Shereshevski-Shere, E., Lasser, L, & Gottesfeld, B. An evaluation of anatomy content and F+ percentage in the Rorschachs of alcoholics, schizophrenics and normals. *Journal of Projective Techniques*, 1953, *17*, 229–233.

Sherman, M. The diagnostic significance of constriction-dilation on the Rorschach. *Journal of General Psychology*, 1955, *53*, 11–19.

Shneidman, E.S. Some relationships between thematic and drawing materials. In E.F. Hammer (Ed.), *The clinical application of projective drawings*. Springfield, IL.: Charles C. Thomas, 1958.

Siegal, R., Rosen, I., & Ehrenreich, G. The natural history of an outcome prediction. *Journal of Projective Techniques*, 1962, *26*, 112–116.

Siegel, E.L. Genetic parallels of perceptual structuralization in paranoid schizophrenia: An analysis by means of the Rorschach technique. *Journal of Projective Techniques*, 1953, *17*, 151–161.

Siegman, A.W. Cognitive, affective, and psychopathological correlates of the Taylor Manifest Anxiety Scale. *Journal of Consulting Psychology*, 1956, *20*, 137–141.

Simpson, C.D., & Vega, A. Unilateral brain damage and patterns of age-corrected WAIS subtest scores. *Journal of Clinical Psychology*, 1971, *27*, 204–208.

Singer, J.L. Delayed gratification and ego development: Implications for clinical and experimental research. *Journal of Consulting Psychology*, 1955, *19*, 259–266.

Singer, J.L. The experience type: Some behavioral correlates and theoretical implications. In M. Rickers-Ovsiankina (Ed.), *Rorschach psychology*. New York: John Wiley & Sons, Inc., 1960.

Singer, J.L., & Herman, J. Motor and fantasy correlates of Rorschach human movement responses. *Journal of Consulting Psychology*, 1954, *18*, 325–331.

Singer, J.L., Meltzoff, J., & Goldman, G.D. Rorschach movement responses following motor inhibition and hyperactivity. *Journal of Consulting Psychology*, 1952, *16*, 359–364.

Singer, J.L., & Spohn, H.E. Some behavioral correlates of Rorschach's experience type. *Journal of Consulting Psychology*, 1954, *18*, 1–9.

Singer, J.L., & Sugarman, D. A note on some projected familial attitudes associated with Rorschach movement responses. *Journal of Consulting Psychology*, 1955, *19*, 117–119.

Singer, J.L., Wilensky, H., & McCraven, V. Delaying capacity, fantasy, and planning ability: A factorial study of some basic ego functions. *Journal of Consulting Psychology*, 1956, *20*, 375–383.

Sinnett, K., & Mayman, M. The Wechsler Adult Intelligence Scale as a clinical diagnostic tool: A review. *Bulletin of the Menninger Clinic*, 1960, *24*, 80–84.

Sloan, W., & Cutts, R.A. Test patterns of defective delinquents on the Wechsler-Bellevue test. *American Journal of Mental Deficiency*, 1945, *50*, 95–97.

Small, L. *Neuropsychodiagnosis in psychotherapy*. New York: Brunner/Mazel, 1973.

Smith, A. Ambiguities in concepts and studies of "brain damage" and "organicity." *Journal of Nervous and Mental Disease*, 1962, *135*, 311–326.

Smith, A. Intellectual functions in patients with lateralized frontal tumours. *Journal of Neurology, Neurosurgery, and Psychiatry*, 1966, *29*, 52–59.

Smith, A. Dominant and nondominant hemispherectomy. In M. Kinsbourne & W.L. Smith (Eds.), *Hemispheric disconnection and cerebral function*. Springfield, IL.: Charles C. Thomas, 1974.

Smith, H.H. Jr., & Smith, L.S. WAIS functioning of cirrhotic and non-cirrhotic alcoholics. *Journal of Clinical Psychology*, 1977, *33*, 309–313.

Smith, W.L. Dynamics of cortical function assessment. In W.L. Smith & M.J. Philippus (Eds.), *Neuropsychological testing in organic brain dysfunction*. Springfield, IL.: Charles C. Thomas, 1969.

Smith, W.L., & Philippus, M.J. (Eds.). *Neuropsychological testing in organic brain dysfunction*. Springfield, IL.: Charles C. Thomas, 1969.

Solkoff, N. Frustration and WISC coding performance among brain-injured children. *Perceptual and Motor Skills*, 1964, *18*, 54.

Solkoff, N., & Chrisien, G. Frustration and perceptual-motor performance. *Perceptual and Motor Skills*, 1963, *17*, 282.

Sommer, R., & Sommer, D. Assaultiveness and two types of Rorschach color responses. *Journal of Consulting Psychology*, 1958, *22*, 57–62.

Spence, J.T. Patterns of performance on WAIS Similarities in schizophrenic, brain damaged and normal subjects. *Psychological Reports*, 1963, *13*, 431–436.

Spielberger, C.D. Anxiety as an emotional state. In C.D. Spielberger (Ed.), *Anxiety: Current trends in theory and research* (Vol. II). New York: Academic Press, 1972.

Spivack, G., Levine, M., & Sprigle, H. Intelligence test performance and the delay function of the ego. *Journal of Consulting Psychology*, 1959, *23*, 428–431.

Stavrianos, B.K. Can projective test measures aid in the detection and differential diagnosis of reading deficit? *Journal of Personality Assessment*, 1971, *35*, 80–91.

Sternberg, D., & Levine, A. An indicator of suicidal ideation on the Bender Visual-Motor Gestalt Test. *Journal of Projective Techniques and Personality Assessment*, 1965, *29*, 377–379.

Stevens, D.A., Boydstun, J.A., Dykman, R.A., Peters, J.E., & Sinton, D.W. Presumed minimal brain dysfunction in children: Relationship to performance on selected behavioral tests. *Archives of General Psychiatry*, 1967, *16*, 281–285.

Stone, N.M., & Schneider, R. E. Concurrent validity of the Wheeler signs of homosexuality in the Rorschach: P(Ci/Rj). *Journal of Personality Assessment*, 1975, *39*, 573–579.

Story, R.I. The Revised Bender-Gestalt and male alcoholics. *Journal of Projective Techniques*, 1960, *24*, 186–193.

Strother, C.R. The performance of psychopaths on the Wechsler-Bellevue test. *Proceedings of the Iowa Academy of Science*, 1944, *51*, 397–400.

Suczek, R.F., & Klopfer, W.G. Interpretation of the Bender Gestalt Test: The associative value of the figures. *American Journal of Orthopsychiatry*, 1952, *22*, 62–75.

Sundberg, N.D. The practice of psychological testing in clinical services in the United States. *American Psychologist*, 1961, *16*, 79–83.

Swensen, C.H. Empirical evaluations of human figure drawings: 1957–1966. *Psychological Bulletin*, 1968, *70*, 20–44.

Symmes, J., & Rapaport, J. Unexpected reading failure. *American Journal of Orthopsychiatry*, 1972, *42*, 82–91.

Symonds, P.M. *The dynamics of human adjustment*. New York: Appleton-Century-Crofts, 1946.

Talkington, L., & Reed, K. An evaluation of Rorschach indicators of psychosis in mentally retarded. *Journal of Projective Techniques and Personality Assessment*, 1969, *33*, 474–475.

Taulbee, E.S. The relationship between Rorschach flexor and extensor M responses and the MMPI and psychotherapy. *Journal of Projective Techniques*, 1961, *25*, 477–479.

Taulbee, E.S., & Sisson, B.D. Rorschach pattern analysis in schizophrenia: A cross-validation study. *Journal of Clinical Psychology*, 1954, *10*, 80–82.

Thiesen, J.W. A pattern analysis of structural characteristics of the Rorschach test in schizophrenia. *Journal of Consulting Psychology*, 1952, *16*, 365–370.

Thompson, D.W. *Psychology in clinical practice*. New York: World Publishing, 1965.

Tolor, A. A comparison of the Bender-Gestalt Test and the Digit Span test as measures of recall. *Journal of Consulting Psychology*, 1956, *20*, 305–309.

Tolor, A. Further studies on the Bender-Gestalt Test and the Digit-Span test as measures of recall. *Journal of Clinical Psychology*, 1958, *14*, 14–18.

Tolor, A. The graphomotor techniques. *Journal of Projective Techniques and Personality Assessment*, 1968, *32*, 222–228.

Tolor, A., & Schulberg, H. *An evaluation of the Bender-Gestalt test*. Springfield, IL.: Charles C. Thomas, 1963.

Towbin, A.P. Hostility in Rorschach content and overt aggressive behavior. *Journal of Abnormal and Social Psychology*, 1959, *58*, 312–316.

Tucker, J.E., & Spielberg, M. Bender-Gestalt Test correlates of emotional depression. *Journal of Consulting Psychology*, 1958, *22*, 56. (Abstract)

Ullman, L.P., & Krasner, L. *A psychological approach to abnormal behavior* (2nd ed.). Englewood Cliffs, N.J.: Prentice-Hall, 1975.

Urban, W.H. *The Draw-A-Person catalogue for interpretive analysis*. Los Angeles: Western Psychological Services, 1963.

Vane, J., & Eisen, V. The Goodenough Draw-A-Man Test and signs of maladjustment in kindergarten children. *Journal of Clinical Psychology*, 1962, *18*, 276–279.

Vinson, D.B. Responses to the Rorschach test that identify schizophrenic thinking, feeling, and behavior. *Journal of Clinical Experimental Psychopathology*, 1960, *21*, 34–40.

Waehner, T.S. Interpretation of spontaneous drawings and paintings. *Genetic Psychology Monographs*, 1946, *33*, 3–70.

Wagner, E.E. The interaction of aggressive movement responses and anatomy responses on the Rorschach in producing anxiety. *Journal of Projective Techniques*, 1961, *25*, 212–215.

Wagner, E.E. Structural analysis: A theory of personality based on projective techniques. *Journal of Personality Assessment*, 1971, *35*, 422–435.

Wagner, E.E. Diagnosis of conversion hysteria: An interpretation based on structural analysis. *Journal of Personality Assessment*, 1973, *37*, 5–15.

Wagner, E.E., & Slemboski, C.A. Construct validation of Piotrowski's interpretation of the Rorschach shading response. *Journal of Projective Techniques and Personality Assessment*, 1969, *33*, 343–344.

Wagner, E.E., & Wagner, C.F. Smiliar Rorschach patterning in three cases of anorexia nervosa. *Journal of Personality Assessment*, 1978, *42*, 426–432.

Walker, R.E., & Spence, J.T. Relationship between Digit Span and anxiety. *Journal of Consulting Psychology*, 1964, *28*, 220–223.

Wallen, R. The nature of color shock. *Journal of Abnormal and Social Psychology*, 1948, *43*, 346–356.

Waller, P. A comparison of shading responses obtained with two Rorschach methodologies from psychiatric and non-psychiatric subjects. *Journal of Consulting Psychology*, 1960, *24*, 43–45. (a)

Waller, P. The relationship between the Rorschach shading response and other indices of anxiety. *Journal of Projective Techniques*, 1960, *24*, 211–217. (b)

Warren, H.C. *Dictionary of psychology*. Boston: Houghton Mifflin, 1934.

Watkins, J.G., & Stauffacher, J.C. An index of pathological thinking in the Rorschach. *Journal of Projective Techniques*, 1952, *16*, 276–286.

Watson, C.G. WAIS profile patterns of hospitalized brain-damaged and schizophrenic patients. *Journal of Clinical Psychology*, 1965, *21*, 294–296.

Watson, C.G., Thomas, R.W., Andersen, D., & Felling, J. Differentiation of organics from schizophrenics at two chronicity levels by use of the Reitan-Halstead organic test battery. *Journal of Consulting and Clinical Psychology*, 1968, *32*, 679–684.

Waugh, K.W., & Bush, W.J. *Diagnosing learning disorders*. Columbus, OH.: Merrill, 1971.

Webster's new world dictionary. New York: World, 1976.

Wechsler, D. *The measurement of adult intelligence* (3rd ed.). Baltimore: Williams & Wilkins, 1944.

Wechsler, D. *The measurement and appraisal of adult intelligence* (4th ed.). Baltimore: William & Wilkins, 1958.

Wechsler, D., & Jaros, E. Schizophrenic patterns on the WISC. *Journal of Clinical Psychology*, 1965, *21*, 288–291.

Weider, A. Effects of age on the Bellevue Intelligence Scales in schizophrenic patients. *Psychiatric Quarterly*, 1943, *17*, 337–346.

Weider, A., & Noller, P. Objective studies of children's drawings of human figures. II. Sex, age, intelligence. *Journal of Clinical Psychology*, 1953, *9*, 20–23.

Weiner, I.B. Cross-validation of a Rorschach checklist associated with suicidal tendencies. *Journal of Consulting Psychology*, 1961, *25*, 312–315. (a)

Weiner, I.B. Three Rorschach scores indicative of schizophrenia. *Journal of Consulting Psychology*, 1961, *25*, 436–439. (b)

Weiner, I.B. Rorschach tempo as a schizophrenic indicator. *Perceptual and Motor Skills*, 1962, *15*, 139–141.

Weiner, I.B. Pure C and color stress as Rorschach indicators of schizophrenia. *Perceptual and Motor Skills*, 1964, *18*, 484.

Weiner, I.B. *Psychodiagnosis in schizophrenia*. New York: John Wiley & Sons, Inc., 1966.

Weiner, I.B. Approaches to Rorschach validation. In M. Rickers-Ovsiankina (Ed.), *Rorschach psychology* (2nd ed.). New York: Krieger, 1977.

Weiner, I.B., & Exner, J.E. Rorschach indices of disordered thinking in patient and nonpatient adolescents and adults. *Journal of Personality Assessment*, 1978, *42*, 339–343.

Weissman, S.L., & Roth, A. *Psychodynamic aspects of the Bender-Gestalt Visual Motor Test*. White Plains, N.Y.: Postgraduate Center for Mental Health, 1965. (Mimeograph)

Wenck, L.S. *House-Tree-Person drawings: An illustrated diagnostic handbook*. Los Angeles: Western Psychological Services, 1977.

Werner, H. Perceptual behavior of brain-injured, mentally defective children: An experimental study by means of the Rorschach technique. *Genetic Psychology Monographs*, 1945, *31*, 51–110.

Wheeler, W.M. An analysis of Rorschach indices of male homosexuality. *Journal of Projective Techniques*, 1949, *13*, 97–126.

White, M.A., & Schreiber, H. Diagnosing "suicidal risks" on the Rorschach. *Psychiatry Quarterly Supplement*, 1952, *26*, 161–189.

White, R.B., Jr. Variations of Bender-Gestalt constriction and depression in adult psychiatric patients. *Perceptual and Motor Skills*, 1976, *42*, 221-222.

Wiener, G. Neurotic depressives' and alcoholics' oral Rorschach percepts. *Journal of Projective Techniques*, 1956, *20*, 453–455.

Wiener, G. The Bender Gestalt Test as a predictor of minimal neurologic deficit in children eight to ten years of age. *Journal of Nervous and Mental Disease*, 1966, *143*, 275–280.

Wiens, A.N., Matarazzo, J.D., & Gaver, K.D. Performance and verbal IQ in a group of sociopaths. *Journal of Clinical Psychology*, 1959, *15*, 191–193.

Wildman, R.W. The relationship between knee and arm joints on human figure drawings and paranoid trends. *Journal of Clinical Psychology*, 1963, *19*, 460–461.

Williams, M. An experimental study of intellectual control under stress and associated Rorschach factors. *Journal of Consulting Psychology*, 1947, *11*, 21–29.

Windle, C. Psychological tests in psychopathological prognosis. *Psychological Bulletin*, 1952, *49*, 451–482.

Wittenborn, J.R., & Holzberg, J.D. The Wechsler-Bellevue and descriptive diagnosis. *Journal of Consulting Psychology*, *15*, 325–329.

Wolff, W. *Personality of the pre-school child*. New York: Grune & Stratton, 1946.

Wolk, R.L. Projective drawings (H-T-P-P) of aged people. In J.N. Buck & E.F. Hammer (Eds.), *Advances in the House-Tree-Person technique: Variations and applications*. Los Angeles: Western Psychological Services, 1969.

Wolman, B.B. Schizophrenia in childhood. In B.B. Wolman (Ed.), *Manual of child psychopathology*. New York: McGraw-Hill, 1972.

Wolman, B.B. (Ed.). *Clinical diagnosis of mental disorders: A handbook*. New York: Plenum Publishing Corp., 1978.

Woltmann, A.G. The Bender Visual-Motor Gestalt Test. In L. Abt & L. Bellak (Eds.), *Projective psychology*. New York: Knopf, 1950.

Wysocki, A.C., & Wysocki, B.A. Human figure drawings of sex offenders. *Journal of Clinical Psychology*, 1977, *33*, 278–284.

Wysocki, B.A., & Whitney, E. Body image of crippled children as seen in Draw-a-Person test behavior. *Perceptual and Motor Skills*, 1965, *21*, 499–504.

Yamahiro, R.S., & Griffith, R.M. Validity of two indices of sexual deviancy. *Journal of Clinical Psychology*, 1960, *16*, 21–24.

Yates, A.J. The use of vocabulary in the measurement of intellectual deterioration—a review. *Journal of Mental Science*, 1956, *102*, 409–440.

Zelen, S.L. Rorschach patterns in three generations of a family. In Klopfer et al., *Developments in the Rorschach technique, Vol. III: Aspects of personality structure*. New York: Harcourt Brace Jovanovich, 1970.

Zimmerman, I.L., & Woo-Sam, J.M. *Clinical interpretation of the Wechsler Adult Intelligence Scale*. New York: Grune & Stratton, 1973.

Zimmerman, J., & Garfinkle, L. Preliminary study of the art productions of the adult psychotic. *Psychiatric Quarterly*, 1942, *16*, 313–318.

Zimmerman, S.F., Whitmyre, J. W., & Fields, F.R.J. Factor analytic structure of the WAIS in patients with diffuse and lateralized cerebral dysfunction. *Journal of Clinical Psychology*, 1970, *26*, 462–465.

Zolik, E.S. A comparison of the Bender Gestalt reproductions of delinquents and non-delinquents. *Journal of Clinical Psychology*, 1958, *14*, 24–26.